Lantern Presents

The Vegan Family Cookbook

Brian P. McCarthy

Lantern Books • New York
A Division of Booklight Inc.

2006
Lantern Books
One Union Square West, Suite 201
New York, NY 10003

Printed in Canada

Cover and interior design by Josh Hooten

Library of Congress Cataloging-in-Publication Data

McCarthy, Brian P., 1965-
The Lantern vegan family cookbook / Brian P. McCarthy.
p. cm.
Includes index.
ISBN 1-59056-087-6 (alk. paper)
1. Vegan cookery. I. Lantern Books. II. Title.
TX837.M2368 2005
641.5'636—dc22
2005023433

Lantern Books has elected to print this title on Enviro Natural, a 100% post-consumer recycled paper, processed chlorine-free. As a result, we have saved the following resources:

102 trees, 4,620 lbs of solid waste, 43,546 gallons of water,
59,010,989 BTUs of energy, 9,029 lbs of net greenhouse gases

As part of Lantern Books' commitment to the environment we have joined the Green Press Initiative, a nonprofit organization supporting publishers in using fiber that is not sourced from ancient or endangered forests. For more information, visit www.greenpressinitiative.org.

Table of Contents

Acknowledgments

To my beautiful wife!
I would like to thank my wife, Karen. She inspired our family to our healthier vegan diet many years ago. Without her there would be no *Lantern Vegan Family Cookbook*. Karen raised the quality of this cookbook to the publishing level by dedicating her limited personal time to countless hours of editing the recipes and providing input on them. She also found time to create some of the more challenging and tasty recipes like the chocolate and white cake. Thank you, "co-author" Karen Davis McCarthy—you never doubted this project!

To my younger son!
Here is a quote from my younger son: "The Broccoli Cauliflower Soup is disgusting, hideous, and gruesome. The worst soup I have ever tasted. No one in their right mind would like it. Its texture is terrible." Thank you, son, for being one of the main recipe testers and for your honest opinions on my cooking. A cook often has a clouded vision of his own cooking and you were always there to speak the truth!

To my older son!
Thank you for your help in organizing this book. You have a great talent for writing and finding ways to organize thoughts on paper. You have also helped me test and taste many recipes. Thank you for always having encouraging words for me!

Welcome!

Some everyday events are taken for granted until you switch to a vegan diet. Mom can no longer share her homemade pecan pie at a family gathering, and Dad doesn't get waffles for breakfast. The kids can't have "normal" cake at their birthday parties or make cookies with their friends. Dinner is brown rice, tofu and salad. Lunch is PB & J, and breakfast is cold cereal. Forget about having friends over for dinner.

My family and I felt this way ten years ago, when my wife and I, after learning about the health drawbacks of the standard American diet, went vegan—and took the kids with us. Suddenly, even though I was a professional cook, I realized I didn't know how to make a good meal for my family. We were all going hungry for "real food." That's when I started this cookbook.

Now, after developing and testing hundreds of recipes, I'm proud to say that living vegan could hardly be easier. Karen's mom makes pizza for grandpa, my mom serves the Moroccan red lentil soup to guests, and Aunt Kathy's summer parties wouldn't be complete without limeade. The chocolate cake is a birthday favorite, and when the kids' friends come knocking, out come the expected chewy oatmeal cookies. Breakfast favorites at our house are lemon poppy seed muffins, sourdough pancakes, and blueberry crepes for special occasions. I have even used these recipes at work. The banana bread is bakery quality, and the fresh herb and garlic pasta is a hit even with non-vegetarians. I'm delighted to present these familiar and delicious dishes that I hope will help make your diet as fulfilling as it should be.

Snacks & Dips

Breadsticks

Yield: 16

1 16-oz. store-bought raw pizza dough or homemade pizza dough (p. 209)
3 Tbs. light olive oil
2 tsp. garlic
2 tsp. basil
¼ tsp. salt

* Roll pizza dough out onto a lightly oiled cookie sheet.

1. Brush the dough with oil.
2. Sprinkle garlic, basil, and salt on dough.
3. Cut into 16 strips.
4. Let rise on counter until doubled in size.
5. Preheat oven to 375°F.
6. Bake for 8 minutes or until done.

A batch of marinara sauce would be great for dipping (see p. 168).

Garbanzo Bean Nuts

Yield: 1½ cups

1 15-oz. can garbanzo beans, drained and rinsed
1 Tbs. light olive oil
2 Tbs. soy sauce*

*Substitute Bragg liquid aminos if you prefer.

*   Preheat oven to 350°F.

1.   Combine all ingredients.
2.   Spread out evenly in a baking dish.
3.   Bake for 1 hour or until beans are crunchy, stirring every 15 minutes.

Variation: SOYBEAN NUTS
Substitute cooked soybeans for the garbanzo beans.

Garlic-Rubbed Baguette

Yield: 9 pieces

1 16-inch baguette
⅓ cup margarine, softened
1 tsp. garlic
1 tsp. oregano
1 tsp. basil
⅛ tsp. salt

*   **Preheat oven to 350°F.**

1.   In a small bowl mix margarine, garlic, oregano, basil, and salt.
2.   On a diagonal, cut baguette into 9 slices.
3.   Spread margarine mixture on both sides of each slice of bread.
4.   Place baguette on a cookie sheet.
5.   Bake for 5–7 minutes.

Variation: CLASSIC-STYLE BAGUETTE
For garlic, oregano, and basil, substitute 1 tsp.
each parsley, sage, ground rosemary, and thyme.

**A great addition to your
favorite Italian dish.**

Popcorn with Yeast Flakes

Yield: 1 large bowl

½ cup popcorn kernels
¼ cup light olive oil
¼ cup nutritional yeast flakes
salt to taste (about ½ tsp.)

1. Pop the popcorn.
2. Mix popcorn with oil and yeast flakes.
3. Add salt to taste.

Nutritional yeast flakes add a cheesy flavor.

Quesadillas

Yield: 4 servings

4 large flour tortillas
1 onion, julienne cut
2 bell peppers, julienne cut
2 Tbs. light olive oil

2 cups shredded cheddar or Monterey jack
   vegan cheese
1 4-oz. can diced green chilies

* Preheat griddle or skillet to 375°F, or choose the medium heat setting on your stove.
* Preheat oven to 160°F.

1. In a 2-quart saucepan, sauté the onions and peppers in the oil until tender.
2. Lay one flour tortilla flat on the preheated griddle. Place ¼ of the onions, peppers, cheese, and green chilies on the tortilla. Grill until cheese starts to melt.
3. Fold in half and grill on each side for 1 minute.
4. Place in a 160° oven to keep warm while you make the remaining quesadillas.
5. Cut each quesadilla into 4 wedges and serve.

Feel free to add or subtract any ingredients you like. Canned re-fried beans, black beans, olives and tomatoes are a few good options.

Roasted Chestnuts

Yield: 4 servings

1 pound chestnuts

*   **Preheat oven to 375°F.**

1. Cut a small X on each chestnut, making sure to pierce the outer shell. This will keep them from exploding in the oven.
2. Place chestnuts on a baking sheet.
3. Roast in oven for 20 minutes, or until outer shell curls up where the X was made.
4. Eat roasted chestnuts while still warm.

> **Look for fresh and local chestnuts to insure full flavor.**

Taquitos

Yield: 18

3 medium potatoes, peeled and quartered
½ onion, diced
2 Tbs. light olive oil
12 oz. vegan chorizo
1 tsp. salt

18 6-inch corn tortillas
¼ cup light olive oil

* **Preheat oven to 350°F.**

1. Boil potatoes until soft, about 15–20 minutes.
2. Drain off water and mash the potatoes. Set aside.
3. In a 3-quart saucepan, sauté the onions in the oil until tender.
4. Add the chorizo, salt, and mashed potatoes to the sautéed onions. Heat until hot.
5. Soften the tortillas.*
6. Divide filling between the 18 tortillas, about ¼ cup each, and roll up.
7. Place rolled-up tortillas in a baking dish.
8. Bake, covered, for 7 minutes.

*You will need to soften the tortillas so they will roll up without cracking. Lightly brush each side of each tortilla with oil, then heat the oiled tortillas slightly. You can do this by microwaving a stack of 6 at a time for about 30 seconds, grilling them lightly on a hot flat surface such as a griddle or skillet, or placing them on a cookie sheet in a preheated 375° oven until warm.

Taquitos are rolled corn tortillas made with assorted fillings. They make a nice snack or entrée.

Chorizo Bean Dip

Yield: 4 cups

2 12-oz. cans refried beans
12 oz. vegan chorizo
1 4-oz. can diced green chilies

1. In a 3-quart saucepan, heat up beans, chorizo, and green chilies.
2. Serve warm.

For a party, place dip in a serving bowl in the center of a large platter. Then arrange different-flavored tortilla chips around the bowl.

Guacamole

Yield: 2 cups

2 ripe avocados, peeled and pitted
1 tomato, diced
¼ cup chopped cilantro (optional)
2 Tbs. lemon juice
½ tsp. garlic
¼ tsp. salt

1. Dice or mash avocado.
2. In a small bowl, combine remaining ingredients with avocado.

Chips, burritos, enchiladas, sandwiches, and wraps are so much better with guacamole!

Hummus

1 15-oz. can garbanzo beans
2 Tbs. lemon juice
2 Tbs. water
1 Tbs. sesame butter

1 Tbs. light olive oil*
1 tsp. onion powder
½ tsp. garlic (optional)
½ tsp. salt

*Substitute sesame oil if you prefer.

1. Drain and rinse beans.
2. Place beans with remaining ingredients into a food processor. Process until smooth.

Variation: GARDEN HUMMUS
To prepared hummus, add ¼ cup each of shredded carrot, shredded zucchini, diced red bell pepper, and chopped cilantro.

Variation: GREEK HUMMUS
To prepared hummus, add ¼ cup chopped olives, ¼ cup diced green onions, and 1 diced tomato.

Variation: SUN-DRIED TOMATO HUMMUS
Boil ¼ cup sun-dried tomatoes for 5 minutes. (If you are using canned sun-dried tomatoes in oil, omit this step.) Drain off water. While processing hummus in food processor, add the sun-dried tomatoes.

Variation: BLACK BEAN HUMMUS
Substitute canned black beans for the garbanzo beans.

Use hummus as a spread on baguettes, pita bread, crackers, sandwiches and wraps. Also makes a great dip for vegetable sticks, chips, or crackers.

Hot Salsa

Yield: 2 cups

12 serranos, chopped
6 habaneros, chopped
2 tomatoes, chopped
½ onion, chopped
1 4-oz. can jalapeños, with liquid
½ cup fresh carrot juice
½ bunch cilantro, chopped
¼ cup lime juice

1 Tbs. red pepper flakes
1½ tsp. balsamic vinegar
1½ tsp. garlic
1½ tsp. chili powder
1½ tsp. cayenne pepper
¼ tsp. salt

*   **Preheat oven to 425°F.**

1. Place chopped serranos, habaneros, tomatoes, and onion in roasting pan.
2. Bake, uncovered, for 30 minutes, stirring every 10 minutes.
3. Place roasted ingredients and remaining ingredients in a food processor or blender.
4. Process until desired texture.

A full-flavored, very hot salsa!

Mild Salsa

Yield: 4 cups

2 tomatoes, diced
½ onion, diced
½ cup chopped cilantro
¼ cup lemon juice
½ tsp. garlic
salt to taste (about ½ tsp.)

1. In a small bowl, combine all ingredients.
2. Add salt to taste.
3. Chill before serving.

Variation: MEDIUM SALSA
Add 1 or 2 Tbs. diced canned jalapeños.

For a gourmet touch, use 1 red tomato and 1 yellow tomato.

Pineapple Salsa

Yield: 2 cups

1 20-oz. can crushed pineapple, drained
1 small red bell pepper, diced
½ small white onion, diced
½ bunch cilantro, chopped
1 or 2 fresh serranos, minced (optional)
¼ cup lemon or lime juice

2 Tbs. seasoned rice vinegar
¼ tsp. salt

Place all ingredients in a food processor or blender, and process until desired texture.

A refreshing fruit salsa to serve with your next Mexican dish.

Salsa Verde

2 12-oz. cans whole tomatillos, drained
1 4-oz. can diced green chilies
½ cup chopped cilantro
½ red bell pepper, diced
½ small white onion, diced
¼ cup lemon or lime juice

1 tsp. garlic
salt to taste (about ½ tsp.)

1. Place all ingredients in a food processor except salt. Process until desired texture.
2. Add salt to taste.

A flavorful salsa that adds a festive color to your party.

Spinach Dip

Yield: 8 servings

12⅓ oz. silken tofu (about 1½ cups)
1 package dry onion soup mix (1 oz.)
½ cup vegan mayonnaise
1 10-oz. package frozen spinach, thawed
    and well drained

1 8-oz. can water chestnuts, diced
½ cup green onions, diced (optional)

1. In a food processor, blend the tofu, onion soup mix, mayonnaise, and spinach until desired smoothness.
2. Place mixture into a large bowl and stir in the water chestnuts and green onions.
3. Chill before serving.

This party dish should chill at least 2 hours before serving.

Tofu Pâté

Yield: 2 cups

16 oz. firm tofu, drained and rinsed
2 celery ribs, minced
½ small white onion, minced
½ cup vegan mayonnaise
1½ Tbs. lemon juice
1 Tbs. yellow mustard

¾ tsp. salt
½ tsp. garlic
½ tsp. onion powder
⅛ tsp. ground black pepper

1. Place tofu in a large, dry, clean dish towel. Squeeze out excess water.
2. Place tofu in a large bowl and mix with remaining ingredients.
3. Place tofu pâté in a food processor for a smoother texture if desired.

This spread is nice for dipping vegetables or crackers in, or use it as a sandwich spread.

Soups

(Hearty and Broth)

Hearty

Broth

Butternut Ginger Soup

Yield: 5 servings

¼ cup light olive oil
1 butternut squash, peeled, seeded, and
   diced
2 carrots, diced
4 ribs celery, diced
½ onion, diced

2 Tbs. minced fresh ginger or 1 tsp. powdered ginger
2 cups vegetable broth*
salt to taste (about 1 tsp.)

*If using the homemade vegetable broth on p. 300, you may need to add salt to this recipe.

1. In a 3-quart saucepan, sauté the squash, carrots, celery, onion, and ginger in the olive oil until tender.
2. Add the vegetable broth and bring to a boil, reduce heat to low, cover and simmer for 40 minutes, stirring occasionally.
3. Puree soup in a blender or food processor. Reheat on stove if necessary.
4. Add salt to taste.

Chili

1 bell pepper

½ onion, chopped

2 Tbs. light olive oil

1 4-oz. can diced green chilies

1 Tbs. chili powder

1 tsp. cumin

½ tsp. garlic (optional)

1 28-oz. can crushed tomatoes

1 15-oz. can black beans, drained and rinsed

1 15-oz. can pinto beans, drained and rinsed

1 cup water

salt to taste (about 1¼ tsp.)

1. In a large pot, sauté the pepper and onion in the oil until tender. Reduce heat to low.
2. Add green chilies, chili powder, cumin, and garlic. Sauté 1 minute.
3. Add tomatoes, beans, and water.
4. Simmer on medium/low heat for 30 minutes, stirring occasionally.
5. Add salt to taste.

Cream of Mushroom Soup

Yield: 3 servings

14 mushrooms, chopped
3 Tbs. light olive oil
3 Tbs. flour
½ tsp. thyme
1½ cups soy milk

½ cup vegetable broth*
salt to taste (about 1 tsp.)

*If using the homemade vegetable broth on p. 300, you may need to add salt to this recipe.

1. In a 3-quart saucepan, sauté the mushrooms in the oil until tender. Reduce heat to low.
2. On reduced heat, add the flour and thyme. Sauté 3 minutes.
3. Turn up heat to medium/high and add soy milk and vegetable broth.
4. Bring to a low boil, stirring constantly.
5. Add salt to taste.

Lentil Soup

1 cup lentils, rinsed
4 cups vegetable broth*
¼ cup tomato paste
2 Tbs. light olive oil
2 ribs celery, diced
1 carrot, diced

¼ onion, diced
2 Tbs. flour
1 tsp. garlic
¼ tsp. thyme
pinch of cayenne, optional
salt to taste (about 2 tsp.)

*If using the homemade vegetable broth on p. 300, you may need to add salt to this recipe.

1. In a 3-quart saucepan, combine lentils and vegetable broth. Bring to a boil, reduce heat to low, cover, and simmer for 1 hour or until lentil are tender.
2. In a 2-quart saucepan, sauté the celery, carrot, and onions in the oil until tender. Reduce heat to low.
3. On reduced heat, add the flour, garlic, thyme, and cayenne and continue to sauté for 2 minutes.
4. Add sautéed vegetables and tomato paste to the cooked lentils.
5. Simmer for 5 minutes.
6. Add salt to taste.

Lentil soup adds protein to your diet and makes a meal all by itself.

Moroccan Red Lentil Soup

Yield: 6 servings

4 ribs celery
½ onion
2 Tbs. light olive oil
½ tsp. ginger
½ tsp. cinnamon
½ tsp. turmeric
6 cups vegetable broth*

4 plum tomatoes, diced
1 cup red lentils
1 15-oz. can garbanzo beans, drained and rinsed
1 bunch cilantro, chopped
2 Tbs. lemon juice
salt to taste (about 1 tsp.)

*If using the homemade vegetable broth on p. 300, you may need to add salt to this recipe.

1. In a large pot, sauté celery and onion in the oil until tender.
2. Add ginger, cinnamon, turmeric, vegetable broth, tomatoes, lentils, and garbanzo beans.
3. Bring to a boil, reduce heat to low, cover, and simmer for 45 minutes or until lentils are tender, stirring occasionally.
4. Right before serving, add cilantro and lemon juice.
5. Add salt to taste.

Navy Bean Soup

Yield: 5 servings

1 cup dry small white beans, rinsed
4 cups water
¼ cup light olive oil
1 carrot, diced
½ onion, diced
2 ribs celery, diced
½ tsp. garlic

¼ tsp. black pepper
¼ tsp. thyme
¼ cup flour
¼ cup tomato paste
4 cups vegetable broth*
salt to taste (about 1½ tsp.)

*If using the homemade vegetable broth on p. 300, you may need to add salt to this recipe.

* Soak the beans in the 4 cups of water overnight.

1. Drain and rinse beans and set aside.
2. In a large stockpot, sauté the carrot, onion, and celery in the oil until tender. Reduce heat to low.
3. On reduced heat, add the garlic, pepper, thyme, and flour and sauté 2 minutes.
4. Add tomato paste, vegetable broth, and beans.
5. Heat soup to a near boil, reduce heat to low, cover and simmer for 2 hours or until beans are tender; stirring occasionally.
6. Add salt to taste.

Variation: ITALIAN BEAN SOUP
Omit tomato paste and add 1 tsp. basil and 1 tsp. oregano with other spices.

A classic bean soup.

Potato Leek Soup

Yield: 5 servings

2 potatoes, peeled and ¾-inch dice
1 red bell pepper, diced
2 cups chopped leeks (about ½ leek)
¼ cup olive oil
⅓ cup flour
2 tsp. onion powder

1 tsp. thyme
½ tsp. garlic
¼ tsp. black pepper
2 cups soy milk
1½ cups vegetable broth*
salt to taste (about 1½ tsp.)

*If using the homemade vegetable broth on p. 300, you may need to add salt to this recipe.

1. Place potatoes in boiling water. Boil until soft but not mushy, about 8–10 minutes. Drain off water and set potatoes aside.
2. In a large stockpot, sauté the red bell pepper and the leeks in the olive oil until tender. Reduce heat to low.
3. On reduced heat, add the flour, onion powder, thyme, garlic, and pepper, and continue to sauté for 2 minutes.
4. Add soy milk and vegetable broth. Heat soup to a near boil or until thickened, stirring occasionally.
5. Gently stir in the cooked potatoes.
6. Add salt to taste.

Root Stew with Marjoram

¼ cup light olive oil
1 fennel root, peeled and diced
1 small turnip, diced
3 carrots, diced
3 ribs celery, diced
½ onion, diced
8 mushrooms, sliced
⅓ cup flour

1 bunch fresh marjoram, chopped
½ bunch fresh parsley, chopped
1 tsp. garlic
¼ tsp. ground black pepper
2 cups vegetable broth*
2 cups store-bought mushroom soup
salt to taste (about 2 tsp.)

*If using the homemade vegetable broth on p. 300, you may need to add salt to this recipe.

1. In a large saucepan, sauté the fennel, turnip, carrots, celery, and onion in the olive oil until vegetables are tender. Reduce heat to low.
2. Add the sliced mushrooms, flour, marjoram, parsley, garlic, and black pepper, and continue to sauté for 2 more minutes while on reduced heat.
3. Add the vegetable broth and mushroom soup.
4. Heat on medium/high heat until a near boil and then let simmer on low heat for 5 minutes, stirring occasionally.
5. Add salt to taste.

Fennel root has a slight licorice flavor that blends nicely with the mushrooms in this fall stew.

Split Pea Soup

1 cup green split peas, rinsed
4 cups water
4 cups vegetable broth*
¼ cup light olive oil
1 carrot, diced
3 ribs celery, diced

1 small onion, diced
¼ cup flour
1 tsp. thyme
½ tsp. garlic
¼ tsp. black pepper
salt to taste (about 2 tsp.)

*If using the homemade vegetable broth on p. 300, you may need to add salt to this recipe.

1. In a large stockpot, soak the split peas in the 4 cups of water for 1 hour or overnight. Drain and rinse the split peas.
2. Return the split peas to the stockpot and add the vegetable broth. Bring to a boil, reduce heat to low, cover, and simmer for 1 hour or until peas are tender.
3. In a 3-quart saucepan, sauté the carrot, celery, and onion in the olive oil until tender. Reduce heat to low.
4. On reduced heat, add the flour, thyme, garlic, and black pepper and continue to sauté for 2 minutes.
5. Add sautéed vegetables to the cooked split peas. Bring soup to a boil, reduce heat to low, and simmer for 5 minutes.
6. Add salt to taste.

A high-protein soup.

Adzuki & Peanut Soup

Yield: 6 servings

1 cup dried adzuki beans, rinsed
4 cups water
2 carrots, diced
3 ribs celery, diced
½ onion, diced
1 bell pepper, diced
¼ cup light olive oil

⅓ cup flour
1 tsp. garlic
1 tsp. thyme
¼ tsp. black pepper
4 cups vegetable broth *
salt to taste (about 2 tsp.)
1½ cups roasted peanuts

*If using the homemade vegetable broth on p. 300, you may need to add salt to this recipe.

1. In a large pot, combine water and beans. Bring to a boil, reduce heat to low, and simmer for 1 hour or until beans are tender.
2. Drain off water and set beans aside.
3. In a large pot, sauté the carrots, celery, onions, and bell pepper in the oil until vegetables are tender. Reduce heat to low.
4. On reduced heat, add the flour, garlic, thyme, and black pepper and continue to sauté for 2 minutes.
5. Add the vegetable broth and the reserved cooked beans.
6. Heat soup on medium/high heat until hot and thickened, stirring often.
7. Add salt to taste.
8. Sprinkle peanuts on top right before serving.

A high-protein soup garnished with crunchy peanuts.

Minestrone Soup

2 carrots, diced
3 ribs celery, diced
½ onion, diced
3 Tbs. light olive oil
4 cups vegetable broth*
½ cup uncooked elbow pasta
½ bunch spinach, chopped

1 15-oz. can diced or crushed tomatoes
1 15-oz. can kidney beans, drained and
   rinsed
1½ tsp. basil
1 tsp. oregano
1 tsp. garlic (optional)
salt to taste (about 1½ tsp.)

*If using the homemade vegetable broth on p. 300, you may need to add salt to this recipe.

1. In a large pot, sauté the carrots, celery, and onion in the oil until tender.
2. Add vegetable broth, pasta, spinach, tomatoes, kidney beans, basil, oregano, and garlic.
3. Bring to a boil, stirring often. Reduce heat to low and cover.
4. Let simmer for 15 minutes or until pasta is cooked, stirring occasionally.
5. Add salt to taste.

Minestrone soup can be made with a variety of beans and vegetables.

Miso Soup

½ white onion, small dice
3 cloves garlic, minced
1 small carrot, diced
½ stalk lemon grass, minced
1 Tbs. sesame oil
½ small savory cabbage, small dice
¼ pound cremini mushrooms, sliced

¼ tsp. red pepper flakes, optional
2 Tbs. white miso paste
1 quart mushroom or vegetable broth
½ pound firm tofu, large dice
½ bunch cilantro, chopped
½ bunch green onions, chopped

1. In a large stockpot, sauté the onion, garlic, carrot, and lemon grass with the sesame oil until tender. Reduce heat to low.
2. On reduced heat, add the cabbage, mushrooms, pepper flakes, and miso, and continue to sauté for 2 minutes.
3. Add mushroom broth. Raise heat and bring soup to a boil.
4. Add the tofu, cilantro, and green onion.
5. Simmer for 2 minutes and serve.

This exotic soup leaves a pleasant aroma in the kitchen for hours.

Tortilla Soup

1 small onion, diced
1 green bell pepper, diced
¼ cup light olive oil
1 tsp. chili powder
½ tsp. garlic
3 cups vegetable broth*

1 cup mild salsa (p. 13)
½ cup frozen corn
1 Tbs. cornstarch
salt to taste (about 1 tsp.)
6 6-inch corn tortillas, cut into 8 wedges
each

*If using the homemade vegetable broth on p. 300, you may need to add salt to this recipe.

1. In a 3-quart saucepan, sauté the onions and peppers in the oil until tender. Reduce heat to low.
2. On reduced heat, add the chili powder and garlic and continue to sauté for 2 more minutes.
3. Add the vegetable broth, salsa, corn, and cornstarch. Stir well.
4. Heat soup on medium/high heat until a near boil, then simmer on low heat for 5 minutes, stirring occasionally.
5. Add salt to taste.
6. Gently stir in the tortillas two minutes before serving.

Serve with warm corn bread (see p. 211).

Vegetable Noodle Soup

4 oz. uncooked pasta (ribbon, rotini, or penne)
2 carrots, diced
3 ribs celery, diced
½ onion, diced

3 Tbs. light olive oil
½ tsp. thyme
½ tsp. onion powder
4 cups vegetable broth*
salt to taste (about ¾ tsp.)

*If using the homemade vegetable broth on p. 300, you may need to add salt to this recipe.

1. Cook pasta according to package directions. Drain off water and set pasta aside.
2. In a large saucepan, sauté carrots, celery, and onion in the oil until tender. Reduce heat to low.
3. On reduced heat, add thyme and onion powder. Sauté 1 minute.
4. Turn up heat to medium/high and add vegetable broth. Bring to a near boil.
5. Gently stir in cooked pasta.
6. Add salt to taste.

Vegetable Soup

2 carrots, diced
3 ribs celery, diced
½ onion, diced
3 Tbs. light olive oil
½ tsp. thyme
½ tsp. onion powder

4 cups vegetable broth*
½ cup corn
½ cup peas
½ cup chopped green beans
salt to taste (about ¾ tsp.)

*If using the homemade vegetable broth on p. 300, you may need to add salt to this recipe.

1. In a large saucepan, sauté carrots, celery, and onion in the oil until tender. Reduce heat to low.
2. On reduced heat, add thyme and onion powder. Sauté 1 minute.
3. Turn up heat to medium/high and add vegetable broth, corn, peas, and green beans. Bring to a boil, reduce heat to low, and simmer for 15 minutes.
4. Add salt to taste.

Salads & Dressings

Salads

Dressings

Caesar Salad

Yield: 6 salads

1 bunch romaine
Caesar salad dressing (p. 59)
2 cups croutons (p. 297)
¼ cup vegan parmesan cheese (p. 298)

1. Chop romaine into bite-sized pieces. Drain off as much water from romaine as possible, using a salad spinner if available.
2. Just before mealtime, toss the romaine with desired amount of salad dressing.
3. Top with croutons and vegan cheese.

An all-time favorite.

Cauliflower Basil Salad

Yield: 6 servings

1 head cauliflower, cut into bite-sized pieces
1 bunch basil, stemmed and chopped
1 red bell pepper, julienne cut
½ red onion, julienne cut
1 carrot, shredded
¼ cup rice vinegar

2 Tbs. light olive oil
½ tsp. garlic
salt to taste (about ½ tsp.)
pepper to taste (about ¼ tsp.)

1. In a large bowl, toss all ingredients except salt and pepper.
2. Add salt and pepper to taste.
3. Serve chilled.

Delightfully crunchy.

Cauliflower & Green Olive Salad

Yield: 8 servings

3 cups cooked brown rice,* cooled (p. 90)
4 green onions, chopped (just bottom half
    of onion, not too much green)
2 celery ribs, diced
½ cup sliced green olives

1 cup bite-sized cauliflower pieces
½ green bell pepper, diced
1 cup vegan mayonnaise
1 Tbs. lemon juice
salt to taste (about ¾ tsp.)

*You can substitute white rice if you prefer.

1. In a large bowl, combine all ingredients except salt.
2. Add salt to taste.

Chinese Mandarin Salad

1 bunch romaine, chopped

20 snow pea pods, stems removed

2 11-oz. cans mandarin orange segments, drained

1 15-oz. can whole baby corn, drained

1 8-oz. can sliced water chestnuts, drained

8 oz. ready-to-serve teriyaki tofu, diced*

⅛ cup toasted sesame seeds (p. 299)

1 cup Oriental Sesame Dressing** (p. 61)

*To make your own teriyaki tofu, see p. 295.

**Substitute your favorite store-bought dressing if you prefer.

1. In a large bowl, combine all salad ingredients except dressing.
2. Serve with dressing on the side.

Chinese Sesame Salad

Yield: 5 dinner salads

1 iceberg lettuce, sliced very thin
8 oz. ready-to-serve teriyaki tofu, large
  dice*
1 red bell pepper, minced

½ bunch green onions, chopped
½ bunch cilantro, chopped
½ cup sliced toasted almonds (p. 299)
1 cup Oriental Sesame Dressing (p. 61)

*To make your own teriyaki tofu, see p. 295.

1. In a large bowl, combine lettuce, tofu, bell pepper, green onions, cilantro, and almonds.
2. Just before serving, toss salad with desired amount of Oriental Sesame Dressing.

A family favorite.

Coleslaw

1 small green cabbage, sliced very thin and
    then chopped
1 carrot, shredded

Dressing:
6 oz. silken tofu
¼ cup vegan mayonnaise
¼ cup sugar
¼ cup lemon juice
1 Tbs. apple cider vinegar

1. In a large bowl, combine the green cabbage and carrots.
2. In a blender, blend the tofu, mayonnaise, sugar, lemon juice, and vinegar until smooth.
3. Combine dressing and cabbage mix.

Variation: CARROT GINGER COLESLAW
Omit the cabbage, increase the carrots to 8, add 2 Tbs. fresh minced ginger and one diced red bell pepper.

Variation: MINTED COLESLAW
Add ¼ bunch chopped fresh mint leaves.

Variation: HAWAIIAN COLESLAW
Add 1½ cups canned diced pineapple and 1 diced red bell pepper.

Coleslaw is best if the dressing is tossed with the cabbage just before it is served.

Couscous Corn Salad

Yield: 6–8 servings

3 cups cooked couscous, cooled (p. 107)
2 cups frozen corn, thawed
1 bunch cilantro, chopped
1 bell pepper, diced
½ red onion, diced

¼ cup lemon juice
salt to taste (about ¼ tsp.)

1. In a large bowl, combine couscous, corn, cilantro, bell pepper, onion, and lemon juice.
2. Add salt to taste.
3. Serve chilled.

A hearty salad.

Cucumbers in Vinegar

Yield: 4 servings

2 cucumbers, peeled, seeded, and sliced into ⅓-inch pieces
½ tsp. salt
cold water
½ cup white vinegar, or vinegar of choice

1. In a small bowl, combine cucumbers and salt.
2. Add just enough cold water to cover cucumbers.
3. Gently stir until salt dissolves.
4. Refrigerate 10 minutes.
5. Drain off water and add just enough cold water to almost cover the cucumbers.
6. Add vinegar and serve immediately.

Note: Do not make more than will be eaten in the next hour or two, or else the cucumbers will lose their crispness.

Refreshing and light.

Curry Rice Salad

3 cups cooked white (p. 101) or brown rice
  (p. 90), cooled
1 red or green bell pepper, diced
1 carrot, diced
2 Tbs. diced red onion
½ cup frozen peas (thawed)

½ cup raisins
½ cup vegan mayonnaise
2 Tbs. sesame oil
1 Tbs. sugar
¾ tsp. curry powder
salt to taste (about 1 tsp.)

1. In a large bowl, combine all ingredients except salt.
2. Add salt to taste.

Garden Pasta Salad

Yield: 8 servings

8 oz. uncooked rotini pasta
1 or 2 cups bite-sized broccoli pieces
1 or 2 cups bite-sized cauliflower pieces
1 carrot, shredded
½ red bell pepper, diced
Italian dressing (about ¾ cup, recipe on p. 60)

1. Cook pasta according to package directions. Drain off pasta water. Rinse pasta with cold water and place in a large bowl.
2. Add broccoli, cauliflower, carrot, and red bell pepper.
3. And Italian dressing to taste.
4. Serve chilled.

This crisp salad makes a cool summer treat.

Italian Pasta Salad

Yield: 8 servings

8 oz. uncooked penne pasta
1 6-oz. can button mushrooms
1 6½-oz. can marinated artichoke hearts,
    drained
1 2½-oz. can sliced black olives, drained
1 red bell pepper, large dice

1 carrot, shredded
¾ cup Italian dressing (p. 60)
salt to taste (about ½ tsp.)
pepper to taste (about ¼ tsp.)

1. Cook pasta according to package directions. Drain off pasta water. Rinse pasta with cold water and place in a large bowl.
2. In the large bowl, combine remaining ingredients with the pasta.
3. Add salt and pepper to taste.

Macaroni Salad

8 oz. macaroni pasta or any fun shaped
    pasta
3 ribs celery, minced
½ onion, minced
1 carrot, grated
1 2-oz. jar diced pimientos

½ cup vegan mayonnaise
3 Tbs. sweet or dill relish
1 tsp. yellow mustard
salt to taste (about ½ tsp.)
black pepper to taste (about ¼ tsp.)

1. Cook pasta according to package directions. Drain off pasta water. Rinse pasta with cold water and place in a large bowl.
2. Add celery, onion, carrot, pimientos, mayonnaise, relish, and mustard.
3. Add salt and pepper to taste.
4. Serve chilled.

A favorite picnic salad.

Marinated Cucumber Salad

Yield: 6 servings

2 cucumbers, peeled, quartered longways, and cut into ½-inch slices
2 plum tomatoes, large dice
½ red onion, large dice
4 cloves garlic, minced
½ cup fresh parsley, chopped

Marinade:
¾ cup seasoned rice vinegar
¾ cup light olive oil
2 tsp. salt
¼ tsp. black pepper
1 tsp. sugar

1. Place all prepped vegetable ingredients into a large bowl.
2. In a separate bowl, whisk together the marinade ingredients.
3. Pour marinade over vegetables and gently toss. Place salad in refrigerator for 30 minutes.
4. Drain off most of the marinade and serve.

A refreshing gourmet salad.

Potato Salad

4 medium russet potatoes, or potatoes of
    your choice, peeled and quartered
½ cup vegan mayonnaise
2 ribs celery, small dice
¼ sweet onion, small dice
3 Tbs. sweet or dill relish

1 or 2 Tbs. yellow mustard
salt to taste (about ¾ tsp.)
black pepper to taste (about ⅛ tsp.)

1. Boil potatoes until tender but not mushy (approximately 15 to 20 minutes), drain.
   Cool potatoes on a dinner plate in refrigerator.
2. Once potatoes are cold, dice into ½-inch pieces.
3. In a large bowl, mix potatoes, mayonnaise, celery, onion, relish, and mustard.
4. Add salt and pepper to taste.

No summer picnic would be complete without this classic dish.

Red Potato Salad

Yield: 8 servings

8 medium red potatoes, ½-inch dice (6 cups)

Dressing:
6 oz. silken tofu
½ cup vegan mayonnaise
3 ribs celery, diced
½ onion, diced

¼ cup sweet or dill relish
2 Tbs. yellow mustard
1 Tbs. sugar (optional)
1 2-oz. jar diced pimientos (optional)
salt to taste (about 1 tsp.)
black pepper to taste (about ¼ tsp.)

1. Place diced potatoes in boiling water and boil until tender, being careful not to over-cook, about 8–12 minutes.
2. Once potatoes are done cooking, drain off the water and place potatoes in the refrigerator until cooled.
3. In a blender, blend the mayonnaise and tofu until smooth.
4. Put blended mayonnaise and tofu in a large bowl. Add celery, onion, relish, mustard, sugar, and pimientos.
5. After potatoes are cooled, add them to the dressing and gently toss.
6. Add salt and pepper to taste.

Roasted Vegetable Salad with Marinated Grilled Tofu

Yield: 12 servings

1 green bell pepper, large dice
1 red bell pepper, large dice
½ red onion, large dice
½ white onion, large dice
2 Tbs. sesame oil
¾ tsp. garlic
¾ tsp. onion powder

¼ tsp. thyme
½ tsp. salt
1 pound diced marinated grilled tofu* (p. 293)
6 plum tomatoes, diced into 1-inch cubes
¼ bunch parsley, chopped
3 Tbs. soy sauce**

*Substitute store-bought teriyaki tofu if desired.
**Substitute Bragg liquid aminos if desired.

* Preheat oven to 475°F.

1. In a large bowl, toss together bell peppers, onions, oil, garlic, onion powder, thyme, and salt, then pour onto a cookie sheet.
2. Roast uncovered until browned, about 25 minutes.
3. In a large bowl, toss roasted vegetables, tofu, tomatoes, parsley, and soy sauce.
4. Serve chilled.

A gourmet salad, great for parties.

Seashell Pasta Salad

Yield: 6 servings

8 oz. uncooked seashell pasta (small size if available)
2 ribs celery, diced
1 carrot, shredded
1 tomato, diced
½ cup frozen peas, thawed

1 2¼-oz. can sliced black olives
1 2-oz. jar diced pimientos
¼ cup Italian dressing (p. 60)
salt to taste (about ¾ tsp.)

1. Cook pasta according to package instructions. Drain off pasta water. Rinse pasta with cold water and place in a large bowl.
2. Stir in remaining ingredients except salt.
3. Add salt to taste.

Spaghetti Salad

Yield: 7 servings

8 oz. uncooked spaghetti, broken into 3-inch lengths

1 carrot, 2-inch thin julienne cut

1 rib celery, 2-inch thin julienne cut

1 small zucchini, 2-inch thin julienne cut

1 small red or green bell pepper, 2-inch thin julienne cut

3 Tbs. Italian dressing (p. 60)

salt to taste (about ½ tsp.)

pepper to taste (about ¼ tsp.)

1. Boil pasta according to package directions. Drain off pasta water. Rinse pasta with cold water and place in a large bowl.
2. Add carrot, celery, zucchini, bell pepper, and dressing.
3. Add salt and pepper to taste.

Sweet & Sour Carrot Salad

Yield: 6 servings

4 carrots, shredded
1 5½-oz. can pineapple tidbits
1 red bell pepper, diced
1 Tbs. rice vinegar
3 Tbs. sugar
salt to taste (about ¼ tsp.)

1. In a medium-sized bowl, combine all ingredients except salt.
2. Add salt to taste.

Tabouli Salad

1 cup bulgur
water
1 bunch fresh mint, stems removed and
    leaves chopped
1 bunch fresh parsley, chopped
2 medium tomatoes, diced

½ bunch green onions, chopped
¼ cup lemon juice
¼ cup light olive oil
salt to taste (about ¾ tsp.)
black pepper to taste (about ¼ tsp.)

1. In a large bowl, cover bulgur with cool water. Let soak for 30 minutes to 1 hour or until bulgur is soft. Add more water if needed.
2. While bulgur is soaking, prep mint, parsley, tomatoes, and green onions.
3. After bulgur is soft, drain off any excess water.
4. To the softened bulgur, add the mint, parsley, tomatoes, green onions, lemon juice, and oil.
5. Add salt and pepper to taste.
6. Chill for 1 hour before serving.

Variation: COUSCOUS TABOULI SALAD
Substitute 3 cups cooked and cooled couscous
(p. 107) for the bulgur and water.

A classic refreshing salad.

Three Bean Salad

1 15-oz. can green beans, drained and rinsed

1 15-oz. can kidney beans, drained and rinsed

1 15-oz. can garbanzo beans, drained and rinsed

½ sweet white onion, thin julienne cut

¾ cup Italian dressing (p. 60)

1. In a large bowl, mix beans and onion.
2. Stir in dressing. Refrigerate, stirring occasionally, at least 3 to 4 hours, allowing the beans to absorb the flavor of the dressing.

Tossed Greek Salad

Yield: 8 servings

1 bunch romaine, chopped
1 bunch red leaf, chopped
½ red onion, cut into thin rings
2 tomatoes, cut into 8 wedges each
1 cucumber, peeled, seeded and cut into
   half wheels

1 bell pepper, cut into thin rings
1 cup whole pitted black olives (kalamatas
   are nice)
Vinaigrette (p. 64) or Italian dressing (p. 60)

1. Toss all ingredients, except vinaigrette, in a large bowl.
2. Just before serving, toss salad with desired amount of vinaigrette, or serve dressing on the side.

A nice side salad with Mediterranean meals.

Tossed Green Salad

Yield: 10 side salads

1 head iceberg

1 bunch red leaf

1 bunch romaine

2 carrots, shredded

¼ head red cabbage, small dice

2 tomatoes, cut into 8 wedges each

1 cucumber, sliced

1. Core, wash, chop, and drain the iceberg, red leaf, and romaine. Remove excess water with a salad spinner, if available.
2. In a large bowl, toss the greens with the carrots and cabbage.
3. Place greens in a serving bowl and garnish with tomato wedges and cucumber slices.
4. Other garnishes may include radish flowers, red onion rings, or parsley.

Wild Rice Salad

½ cup wild rice
2 cups water
½ cup brown rice
1 small red or green bell pepper
1 carrot, diced
1 cup frozen peas, thawed

1 Tbs. sesame oil
1 Tbs. soy sauce*
seasoned rice vinegar to taste (about 2 or
    more Tbs.)
salt to taste (about ¼ tsp.)

*Substitute Bragg liquid aminos if desired.

1. In a 3-quart saucepan, bring just the wild rice and water to a boil. Reduce heat to low, cover, and simmer for 45 minutes. Add brown rice, cover, and simmer for 45 more minutes.
2. Cool rice.
3. In a large bowl, combine rice and remaining ingredients except vinegar and salt.
4. Add vinegar and salt to taste.

Caesar Salad Dressing

Yield: 1½ cups

1 cup vegan mayonnaise
2 tsp. light olive oil
2 tsp. vegan Worcestershire sauce
¼ cup lemon juice
1 tsp. black pepper

½ tsp. garlic
½ tsp. salt

In a small bowl, combine all ingredients.

Most Worcestershire sauces contain fish oil or anchovy paste, so check the label.

Italian Dressing

Yield: 1 cup

½ cup light olive oil
¼ cup red wine vinegar
1 tsp. garlic
¼ tsp. oregano
¼ tsp. basil

¼ tsp. parsley flakes
¼ tsp. salt

In a small bowl, whisk together all ingredients.

Variation: CREAMY ITALIAN DRESSING
Add ¼ cup vegan mayonnaise.

Oriental Sesame Dressing

Yield: 1 cup

½ cup vegan mayonnaise
2 Tbs. sesame oil
2 Tbs. lime juice*

1 Tbs. rice vinegar
1 Tbs. soy sauce**

*Substitute lemon juice if desired.
**Substitute Bragg liquid aminos if desired.

In a small bowl, whisk together all ingredients.

A flavorful variation for your next salad.

Thai Dressing

Yield: 2½ cups

1 cup seasoned white or brown rice vinegar
½ cup water
½ cup sweet chili sauce
¼ bunch cilantro, chopped

1 small carrot, shredded
2 Tbs. sesame oil
2 Tbs. soy sauce*
2 Tbs. sugar

*Substitute Bragg liquid aminos if desired.

In a small bowl, whisk together all ingredients.

Variation: FAT-FREE THAI DRESSING
Omit sesame oil.

A colorful and exotic dressing.

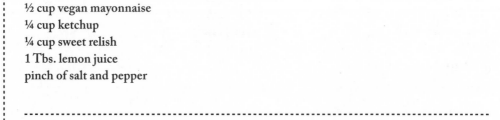

Thousand Island Dressing

Yield: 1 cup

½ cup vegan mayonnaise
¼ cup ketchup
¼ cup sweet relish
1 Tbs. lemon juice
pinch of salt and pepper

In a small bowl, whisk together all ingredients.

Vinaigrette

Yield: 1 cup

½ cup olive oil
2 Tbs. red wine vinegar
¼ cup lemon juice
1 tsp. parsley flakes
½ tsp. oregano
½ tsp. basil

½ tsp. onion powder
½ tsp. garlic
¼ tsp. sugar
¼ tsp. salt
⅛ tsp. black pepper

In a small bowl, combine all ingredients.

Variation: BALSAMIC LIME VINAIGRETTE
Substitute balsamic vinegar for the wine vinegar and lime juice for the lemon juice.

Make your own customized vinaigrette by choosing different and exotic vinegars, oils, and spices.

Chive & Dill Vinaigrette

Yield: 1 cup

½ cup light olive oil
¼ cup balsamic vinegar
2 Tbs. chopped fresh chives
2 Tbs. chopped fresh dill
1½ tsp. lemon juice
¼ tsp. Dijon-style mustard

¼ tsp. salt
⅛ tsp. black pepper

In a small bowl, whisk together all ingredients.

Vegetables

(Roasted, Baked, Sautéed, and Boiled)

Roasted Asparagus

Yield: 5 servings

1 bunch asparagus
1 Tbs. light olive oil
1 Tbs. red wine vinegar
1 tsp. parsley flakes
½ tsp. garlic
½ tsp. oregano

½ tsp. basil
½ tsp. sugar
⅛ tsp. black pepper
salt to taste (about ¼ tsp.)

*   Preheat oven to 425°F.

1. Cut off and discard the bottom 2 inches of each piece of asparagus.
2. In a small bowl, combine all ingredients, except salt.
3. Evenly arrange in a baking dish.
4. Bake, uncovered, for 20 minutes.
5. Add salt to taste.

Roasted Corn

Yield: 4–6 servings

16 oz. frozen corn
½ onion, diced
1 red bell pepper, diced
2 Tbs. light olive oil
½ tsp. garlic
salt to taste (about ½ tsp.)

* Preheat oven to 425°F.

1. In a small bowl, combine all ingredients, except salt.
2. Evenly arrange in a baking dish.
3. Bake, uncovered, for 20 minutes.
4. Add salt to taste.

**The roasting really brings out
the sweetness of the corn.**

Roasted Garlic

Yield: 16 cloves

16 cloves garlic, peeled (1 head)
1 Tbs. light olive oil

*   Preheat oven to 375°F.

1.   In a small bowl, toss garlic with oil.
2.   Evenly arrange garlic in a baking dish.
3.   Bake, covered, for 20 minutes, stirring once after 10 minutes.

You can also roast a whole head of unpeeled garlic. Cut off the top of the head of garlic, exposing the tops of the garlic cloves. Drizzle a small amount of olive oil into the cloves. Completely wrap the garlic head with foil and bake at 375°F until garlic is tender, about 30 minutes. Once the wrapped garlic is cool to the touch, remove foil and squeeze out the roasted garlic cloves though the cut you made earlier, leaving the peel behind.

**Great with potatoes
or fresh bread.**

Roasted Green Beans with Walnuts

Yield: 5 servings

1 pound fresh green beans, stems removed
¼ cup diced walnuts
1 Tbs. light olive oil
1 tsp. rice vinegar
1 tsp. sugar

½ tsp. thyme
salt to taste (about ½ tsp.)

*   Preheat oven to 425°F.

1. In a small bowl, combine all ingredients, except salt.
2. Evenly arrange in a baking dish.
3. Bake, uncovered, for 20 minutes.
4. Add salt to taste.

Roasted Vegetable Medley

Yield: 4 cups

1 fennel root, thin julienne cut
2 small carrots, 3-inch thin julienne cut
½ red onion, thin julienne cut
1 red or green bell pepper, thin julienne cut
1 small zucchini, 3-inch thin julienne cut
2 Tbs. light olive oil

¾ tsp. garlic (optional)
½ tsp. thyme
½ tsp. basil
¼ tsp. red pepper flakes (optional)
salt to taste (about 1 tsp.)

*　　Preheat oven to 475°F.

1. In a large bowl, combine all ingredients.
2. Divide between two large baking dishes.
3. Bake, uncovered, for 20 minutes.
4. Add salt to taste.

Roasted vegetables have a variety of uses. Serve cold on salads, wraps or sandwiches, or serve hot as a side dish or in grilled sandwiches.

Roasted Yam

Yield: 4 servings

1 yam, peeled and julienne cut
1 Tbs. light olive oil
1 Tbs. red wine vinegar
½ tsp. sugar
½ tsp. garlic
½ tsp. oregano

½ tsp. basil
¼ tsp. black pepper
salt to taste (about ½ tsp.)

*   Preheat oven to 425°F.

1. In a small bowl, combine all ingredients, except salt.
2. Evenly arrange in a baking dish.
3. Bake, uncovered, for 25 minutes.
4. Add salt to taste.

Variation: MAPLE GLAZED ROASTED YAM
For sugar, substitute ¼ cup pure maple syrup.

**Serve hot as a side dish,
or cool as a snack.**

Yam Fries

Yield: 5 servings

2 large yams, peeled and julienne cut
2 Tbs. light olive oil
2 Tbs. sugar (optional)
salt to taste (about ½ tsp.)

*   Preheat oven to 375°F.

1. In a medium bowl, combine all ingredients, except salt.
2. Evenly arrange in a baking dish.
3. Bake, uncovered, for 30 minutes.
4. Add salt to taste.

> Date sugar, molasses, or brown sugar can be used in place of the sugar.

Acorn Squash with Molasses

Yield: 2–4 servings

1 acorn squash
2 Tbs. molasses (optional)

* **Preheat oven to 400°F.**

1. Cut squash in half and remove the seeds.
2. Place in a baking dish, flat side down.
3. Bake for 45 minutes or until tender.
4. Remove from oven and scoop the squash out into a bowl.
5. Stir in molasses and serve.

Broccoli & Cauliflower au Gratin

2 cups bite-sized broccoli pieces
2 cups bite-sized cauliflower pieces
2 cups soy milk
¼ cup light olive oil
¼ cup flour
¼ cup nutritional yeast flakes
1 tsp. salt
⅛ tsp. nutmeg

Topping:
1 cup shredded vegan cheddar cheese (4 oz.)
½ cup sliced almonds

*   Preheat oven to 400°F.

1. Place broccoli and cauliflower in boiling water for 3 minutes. Drain off water and set vegetables aside.
2. In a blender, blend soy milk, oil, flour, yeast flakes, salt, and nutmeg until smooth.
3. Place blended ingredients in a 3-quart saucepan. Heat sauce on medium heat until hot and thickened, stirring often.
4. In a 8 x 8-inch baking dish, combine the broccoli, cauliflower, and sauce.
5. Sprinkle cheese and almonds on top.
6. Bake, uncovered, for 10 minutes.

This vegetable dish is satisfying enough to be a dinner entrée.

Butternut Squash with Pumpkin Butter

Yield: 4 servings

1 butternut squash
⅓ cup store-bought pumpkin butter

*   Preheat oven to 375°F.

1. Cut squash in half and remove the seeds.
2. Place in a lightly oiled baking dish, flat side down.
3. Bake, uncovered, for 45 minutes or until tender.
4. Remove from oven and scoop the squash out into a bowl.
5. Stir in pumpkin butter and serve.

Candied Sweet Potatoes

---

4 sweet potatoes, peeled and 1-inch dice
¼ cup brown sugar
1 Tbs. light olive oil
¼ tsp. salt
⅛ tsp. cinnamon
⅛ tsp. nutmeg

---

*   Preheat oven to 375°F.

1. Place diced sweet potatoes in boiling water.
2. Boil until soft but not mushy (about 8–10 minutes). Drain off water.
3. In a medium-sized bowl, toss sweet potatoes with brown sugar, oil, salt, cinnamon, and nutmeg.
4. Place in a baking dish.
5. Bake, uncovered, for 10 minutes.

Variation: CANDIED YAMS
Substitute yams for sweet potatoes.

If you can find vegan marsh-mallows, feel free to top this dish with them right before baking.

Sweet Potatoes & Apples

Yield: 6 servings

2 sweet potatoes, peeled and cut into ¼-inch slabs

2 green apples, peeled, cored and cut into ¼-inch wedges

¼ cup apple juice or water

3 Tbs. brown sugar

1 tsp. cinnamon

3 Tbs. margarine

---

*   Preheat oven to 375°F.

1. Oil a 9 x 13-inch baking dish.
2. Arrange the sweet potatoes on the bottom of the dish.
3. Arrange the apples on top of the sweet potatoes.
4. Pour apple juice or water over the top.
5. Combine sugar and cinnamon in a small bowl.
6. Sprinkle sugar mixture on top of apples.
7. Dot top of dish with margarine.
8. Bake, covered, for 40 minutes or until sweet potatoes are soft.

A fruit and vegetable dish that's always welcome on your dinner table.

Curry Coconut Vegetables

Yield: 6 servings

3 Tbs. sesame oil
1 onion, julienne cut
2 bell peppers, julienne cut
2 carrots, julienne cut
2 cups bite-sized broccoli pieces
2 Tbs. flour

1 Tbs. red curry paste
1 14-oz. can unsweetened coconut milk
salt to taste (about ½ tsp.)

1. Sauté the onions, peppers, carrots, and broccoli in the sesame oil until tender. Reduce heat to low.
2. On reduced heat, add flour and curry paste and continue to sauté for 2 more minutes.
3. Add coconut milk.
4. Simmer for 5 minutes or until hot.
5. Add salt to taste.

Serve over rice or by itself.

Greens with Onions & Garlic

½ onion, diced
2 Tbs. light olive oil
1 bunch collard greens, chopped*
1 tsp. garlic
salt to taste (about ½ tsp.)

*Or substitute any greens you have available, such as Swiss chard or kale.

1. Sauté onions in the oil until tender.
2. Add collard greens and garlic. Continue to sauté until greens are wilted.
3. Add salt to taste.

Sautéed onions and garlic add an excellent flavor to healthy greens.

Miso Kale

Yield: 4 servings

½ onion, diced
2 Tbs. light olive oil
2 Tbs. miso paste
1 bunch kale, rinsed and chopped
½ cup vegetable broth

1. In a large pan, sauté the onions in the oil until tender.
2. Add the miso, kale, and vegetable broth.
3. Continue to cook until the kale is wilted.

Serve this healthy dish by itself, or on top of a bed of couscous or rice.

Oriental Green Beans

Yield: 5 servings

1 lb. fresh green beans, stems removed
3 Tbs. sesame oil
2 Tbs. fresh ginger, minced
¼ cup soy sauce*

*Substitute Bragg liquid aminos if desired.

1. In a large pan, sauté the beans and ginger in the sesame oil until beans are tender.
2. Add soy sauce and sauté for 1 more minute.

**Use fresh local green beans
for the best quality.**

Spanish Brussels Sprouts

Yield: 4–6 servings

1 lb. Brussels sprouts, cut into quarters
1 bell pepper, diced
½ onion, diced
1 Tbs. fresh garlic, minced
3 Tbs. light olive oil
1 tsp. chili powder

1 tsp. oregano
1 10-oz. can crushed tomatoes
salt to taste (about ½ tsp.)

1. In a 2-quart saucepan, sauté the Brussels sprouts, peppers, onion, and garlic in the oil until tender. Reduce heat to low.
2. On reduced heat, add the chili powder and oregano. Continue to sauté for 2 minutes.
3. Add tomatoes and simmer for 5 minutes or until hot.
4. Add salt to taste.

Artichokes

Yield: 4 servings

4 artichokes

1. Bring a large pot of water to a boil.
2. With a sharp knife, cut off the top ½ inch of each artichoke.
3. Place artichokes in boiling water, cover, and cook at a low boil for 30 minutes.

Artichoke leaves are often served with olive oil or melted margarine for dipping. Save the cooked artichoke heart for a salad if desired.

Glazed Baby Carrots

Yield: 4–6 servings

1 pound peeled baby carrots
2 Tbs. sugar
1 tsp. molasses
⅛ tsp. dill

1. Boil carrots for 10 minutes or until tender.
2. Drain off water.
3. Toss carrots with sugar, molasses, and dill.

Who doesn't love these?

Parsnips with Brown Sugar

Yield: 4 servings

2 large parsnips, peeled and cut into bite-sized pieces
2 Tbs. brown sugar
salt to taste (about ¼ tsp.)

1. Boil parsnips 5–10 minutes or until tender. Drain off water.
2. Add brown sugar and salt.

Pickled Beets

Yield: 1 cup

4 medium-sized beets, peeled
¾ cup water
½ cup apple cider vinegar
½ cup sugar
1 tsp. salt

1. Cut beets into ⅛-inch sliced wheels or julienne strips.
2. Place beets and remaining ingredients in a 2-quart saucepan.
3. Bring to a boil, reduce heat to low, cover and simmer for 30 minutes or until beets are soft.
4. Remove beets from heat, place uncovered in refrigerator, and cool for 2 hours. Do not drain off liquid.
5. Refrigerate beets in their liquid, in a sealed container.

Variation: ORANGE BEETS
Substitute 1 cup orange juice for the ¾ cup water.
Reduce the vinegar to ¼ cup.

Homemade pickled beets are easy and delicious.

Side Dishes

(Rice, Potatoes, Pasta, Stuffing, and Beans)

Basmati Rice

Yield: 4 cups cooked rice

1¼ cups basmati rice, rinsed
2½ cups water

1. In a 2-quart saucepan, combine rice and water.
2. Bring to a boil, reduce heat to low, cover, and simmer for 20 minutes or until rice is tender.

Brown Rice

1¼ cups brown rice, rinsed
2½ cups water

1. In a 2-quart saucepan, combine rice and water.
2. Bring to a boil, reduce heat, cover, and simmer for 45 minutes or until rice is tender.

Brown Rice Pilaf

Yield: 4 servings

3 Tbs. light olive oil
½ onion, diced
1 carrot, diced
2 ribs celery, diced
4 mushrooms, sliced
¼ tsp. thyme

¼ tsp. garlic
1 cup brown rice, rinsed
2 cups vegetable broth
salt to taste (about ½ tsp.)

1. In a 3-quart saucepan, sauté the onion, carrot, celery, and mushrooms in the oil until tender. Reduce heat to low.
2. On reduced heat, add the thyme, garlic, and rice, and continue to sauté for 2 minutes.
3. Add vegetable broth.
4. Bring to a boil, reduce heat to low, cover, and simmer for 45 minutes or until rice is tender.
5. Add salt to taste.

Pilaf can be made with a variety of vegetables of your choice.

Coconut Jasmine Rice

Yield: 2 cups cooked rice

1 cup jasmine rice, rinsed
1 14-oz. can unsweetened coconut milk
½ cup water
salt to taste (about ½ tsp.)

1. In a 2-quart saucepan, combine the rice, coconut milk, and water.
2. Slowly bring to a boil, reduce heat to low, cover, and simmer for 25 minutes or until rice is tender.
3. Add salt to taste.

Because this rice tends to burn on the bottom of the pan, heat it up slowly and stir often.

Fried Rice

Yield: 4 servings

1 cup brown rice, rinsed
2 cups vegetable broth*
2 Tbs. sesame oil
6 mushrooms, small dice

2 ribs celery, small dice
1 carrot, small dice
½ onion, small dice
¼ cup soy sauce**

*If using the homemade vegetable broth on p. 300, you may need to add salt to this recipe.
**Substitute Bragg liquid aminos if desired.

1. In a 3-quart saucepan, combine the rice and vegetable broth.
2. Bring to a boil, reduce heat to low, cover, and simmer for 45 minutes or until rice is tender.
3. In a 2-quart saucepan, sauté the mushrooms, celery, carrot, and onion in the sesame oil until tender.
4. Combine the cooked rice, sautéed vegetables, and soy sauce.

Fried rice makes a nice side dish accompanied by a spring roll.

Ginger Rice with Peppers & Soybeans

Yield: 6 servings

1 cup brown rice, rinsed
2 cups vegetable broth*
1 red bell pepper, diced
1 green bell pepper, diced
½ onion, diced

1 carrot, diced
¾ cup frozen soybeans (shelled)
2 Tbs. minced fresh ginger
3 Tbs. sesame oil
¼ cup soy sauce**

*If using the homemade vegetable broth on p. 300, you may need to add salt to this recipe.
**Substitute Bragg liquid aminos if desired.

1. In a 3-quart saucepan, combine the rice and vegetable broth.
2. Bring to a boil, reduce heat to low, cover, and simmer for 45 minutes or until rice is tender
3. In a 2-quart saucepan, sauté the peppers, onion, edamame, and ginger in the oil until tender.
4. Combine cooked rice, sautéed vegetables, and soy sauce.

Hawaiian Rice

Yield: 6 servings

3 Tbs. light olive oil
½ onion, diced
1 red bell pepper, diced
1 cup basmati rice, rinsed
1 14-oz. can unsweetened coconut milk
½ cup water

1 8-oz. can diced pineapple (drained)
salt to taste (about ½ tsp.)

1. In a 2-quart saucepan, sauté the onion and bell pepper in the oil until tender.
2. Add rice, coconut milk, and water.
3. Slowly bring to a boil, reduce heat to low, cover, and simmer for 30 minutes or until rice is tender.
4. Add pineapple.
5. Add salt to taste.

Jasmine Rice

Yield: 4 cups cooked rice

1½ cups jasmine rice, rinsed
2 cups water

1. In a 2-quart saucepan, combine rice and water.
2. Bring to a boil, reduce heat to low, cover, and simmer for 15 minutes or until rice is tender.

Jasmine rice goes well
with Thai food.

Lemon Grass Rice

Yield: 6 servings

2 Tbs. sesame oil
¼ stalk lemon grass, minced
1½ cups basmati rice, rinsed
2½ cups water
salt to taste (about ¼ tsp.)

1. In a 3-quart saucepan, sauté the lemon grass in the oil until tender.
2. Add rice and water, bring to a boil, reduce heat to low, cover, and simmer for 25 minutes or until rice is tender.
3. Add salt to taste.

Fresh lemon grass can be found in the produce section at some local markets.

Mushroom & Wild Rice

Yield: 4 servings

¼ cup wild rice, rinsed
1 cup water
1 carrot, diced
½ onion, diced
6 mushrooms, diced
2 Tbs. light olive oil

½ cup brown rice, rinsed
1¼ cups vegetable broth
½ tsp. garlic
½ tsp. thyme
salt to taste (about 1 tsp.)

1. In a 2-quart saucepan, combine wild rice and water.
2. Bring to a boil, reduce heat to low, cover, and simmer for 45 minutes or until rice is tender.
3. Drain off excess water and set cooked wild rice aside.
4. In a 3-quart saucepan, sauté the carrot, onion, and mushrooms in the oil until tender.
5. Add the cooked wild rice, uncooked brown rice, vegetable broth, garlic, and thyme.
6. Bring to a boil, reduce heat to low, cover, and simmer for 45 minutes or until brown rice is tender.
7. Add salt to taste.

Spanish Rice

Yield: 4 servings

1 cup brown rice, rinsed
2 cups water
2 Tbs. light olive oil
½ onion, diced
1 tsp. chili powder
½ tsp. garlic

½ tsp. oregano
½ tsp. sugar
¼ tsp. cumin
¼ cup water
¼ cup tomato paste
salt to taste (about 1 tsp.)

1. In a 2-quart saucepan, combine rice and 2 cups of water.
2. Bring to a boil, reduce heat to low, cover, and simmer for 45 minutes or until rice is tender.
3. In a separate 2-quart saucepan, sauté the onion until tender. Reduce heat to low.
4. On reduced heat, add chili powder, garlic, oregano, sugar, and cumin, and continue to sauté for 1 minute. Add the ¼ cup water and tomato paste.
5. Add seasoned sautéed onion mix to the cooked rice.
6. Add salt to taste.

A great side dish for your next fiesta.

Sticky Rice

Yield: 4 cups cooked rice

2 cups calrose rice, rinsed
2½ cups water

1. In a 3-quart saucepan, combine rice and water.
2. Bring to a boil, reduce heat to low, cover, and simmer for 25 minutes or until rice is tender.

White Rice

Yield: 4 cups cooked rice

1½ cup long grain white rice, rinsed
3 cups water

---

1. In a 2-quart saucepan, combine rice and water.
2. Bring to a boil, reduce heat, cover, and simmer for 20 minutes or until rice is tender.

French Fries

Yield: 4 servings

4 medium potatoes, peeled and julienne cut
3 Tbs. light olive oil
salt to taste (about 1 tsp.)

*   **Preheat oven to 500°F.**

1. Place cut-up potatoes in a large bowl and toss with oil.
2. Divide between two cookie sheets.
3. Bake for 30 minutes or until crisp.
4. Add salt to taste.

Variation: FRENCH FRIES WITH ROSEMARY
While tossing the potatoes with the oil, add 1 tsp.
ground rosemary.

**What's a veggie burger
without fries?**

Mashed Potatoes

5 medium potatoes, peeled and quartered
8 cups water
¼ cup soy milk
2 Tbs. light olive oil
¼ cup nutritional yeast flakes (optional)

salt to taste (about ½ tsp.)
black pepper to taste (about ¼ tsp.)

1. Place potatoes in boiling water for 20 minutes or until soft.
2. Drain off water.
3. Add the soy milk, olive oil, and yeast flakes.
4. Mash until smooth.
5. Add salt and pepper to taste.

You can add protein and a cheesy flavor to the potatoes with nutritional yeast.

Potato Latkes

3 cups shredded potatoes
1 small onion, diced
½ cup flour
¼ cup light olive oil
1 Tbs. nutritional yeast flakes
1 tsp. baking powder

1 tsp. salt
⅛ tsp. black pepper

*   **Preheat grill to 400°F.**

1. In large bowl, combine all ingredients.
2. Cook latkes like pancakes. Place ⅓ of a cup of mixture on hot grill and flatten.
3. Grill until browned on each side.

**A simple recipe that makes
a nice side dish.**

Roasted Red Potatoes

Yield: 5 servings

6 large red potatoes
3 Tbs. light olive oil
1 tsp. basil
1 tsp. garlic
1 tsp. paprika
½ tsp. thyme

¼ tsp. black pepper
salt to taste (about 1¼ tsp.)

* **Preheat oven to 425°F.**

1. Cut potatoes into 1-inch cubes.
2. Place potatoes in boiling water for 10–15 minutes. Potatoes should be soft but not mushy.
3. Drain off water and place potatoes in a baking dish.
4. Gently toss potatoes with oil, basil, garlic, paprika, thyme, and pepper.
5. Bake, uncovered, for 20 minutes.
6. Add salt to taste.

Serve with country gravy (see p. 280), ketchup, or salsa.

Sweet Potato Polenta

Yield: 4 servings

1 large sweet potato, peeled and large dice
2 cups soy milk
½ tsp. cinnamon
¼ tsp. nutmeg
½ cup polenta (uncooked)

1. In a 2-quart saucepan, boil sweet potato until tender. Drain off water and mash.
2. In a 3-quart saucepan, combine soy milk, cinnamon, and nutmeg. Whisk in polenta. Bring mixture to a boil, reduce heat and simmer for 20 minutes, stirring frequently.
3. Stir in mashed sweet potato.

Variation: YAM POLENTA
Substitute 1 large yam for the sweet potato.

Couscous

Yield: 3 cups cooked couscous

1½ cups water or vegetable broth
1 Tbs. light olive oil
1 cup couscous

1. In a 2-quart saucepan, bring water and oil to a boil. Remove pan from heat.
2. Add couscous. Stir for 30 seconds.
3. Cover and let stand for 6 minutes.
4. Fluff with a fork.

Makes a quick after-school snack.

Indian Couscous

Yield: 4 servings

2 Tbs. light olive oil
½ onion, diced
½ red bell pepper, diced
2 cups vegetable broth
½ cup frozen peas
1 tsp. curry powder

½ tsp. salt
1½ cups couscous

1. In a 3-quart saucepan, sauté the onion and pepper in the olive oil until tender.
2. Add vegetable broth, peas, curry, salt, and cinnamon. Bring to a boil.
3. Remove pan from heat, stir in the couscous, cover, and let stand for 6 minutes.
4. Fluff with a fork.

Herb Stuffing with Almonds

Yield: 6–8 servings

½ onion, diced
4 ribs celery, diced
3 Tbs. light olive oil
1 Tbs. onion powder
1 tsp. sage
1 tsp. thyme

1 tsp. rosemary
½ tsp. salt
2 cups vegetable broth
1¼ lbs sourdough bread, large dice (about 8 cups)
⅗ cup slivered almonds

* Preheat oven to 325°F.

1. In a large pot, sauté the onion and celery in the oil until tender. Reduce heat to low.
2. On reduced heat, add onion powder, sage, thyme, rosemary, and salt. Sauté for 1 minute.
3. Add vegetable broth and simmer for 5 minutes. Remove from heat.
4. Add bread and almonds.
5. Transfer stuffing to a baking dish.
6. Bake, covered, for 30 minutes. For a crispy stuffing, remove the lid for the last 15 minutes.

Variation: APPLE STUFFING

Add 2 peeled and diced green apples with the bread and almonds.

Variation: CORN BREAD STUFFING

Reduce bread to ½ lb. and add 5 cups diced or crumbled corn bread (p. 211).

Variation: CORN BREAD STUFFING WITH APPLE

Reduce bread to ½ lb. Add 2 peeled and diced green apples and 5 cups diced corn bread.

Have plenty of stuffing on hand, because everyone will want more!

Potato Bread Stuffing

Yield: 8 servings

4 medium russet potatoes
1 cup soy milk
5 slices bread of your choice, diced
½ onion, minced
2 ribs celery, minced
1 Tbs. light olive oil

1 tsp. salt
1 tsp. thyme
½ tsp. sage
½ tsp. ground rosemary
½ tsp. onion powder
¼ tsp. black pepper

* **Preheat oven to 400°F.**

1. Bake potatoes until tender, 1 to 1½ hours. Reduce oven heat to 350.
2. Cut potatoes lengthwise and scoop out insides into a large saucepan. Place potato skins in a 9 x 13-inch baking dish and set aside.
3. Mash the potatoes in the large saucepan.
4. Add soy milk, bread, onion, celery, oil, salt, thyme, sage, rosemary, onion powder, and black pepper. Mix well.
5. Fill potato skins with the stuffing.
6. Bake, uncovered, for 45 minutes.

**Potato stuffing served
in potato skins.**

Baked Beans

2½ cups uncooked small white beans, rinsed
8 cups water for overnight soaking
8 cups water for boiling
2 Tbs. light olive oil
½ onion, diced
¼ cup flour
½ cup sugar
¼ cup molasses

1 Tbs. yellow mustard
2 tsp. white vinegar
1 tsp. onion powder
1 tsp. garlic
2 cups vegetable broth
1 4-oz. can tomato paste
salt to taste (about 1 Tbs.)

1. Soak beans in 8 cups water overnight.
2. Drain and rinse beans.
3. Place beans in large stockpot with 8 cups water.
4. Bring to a boil, reduce heat to low, cover, and simmer for 2 hours or until tender.
5. Drain off water and set beans aside.
6. In a large stockpot, sauté onion in the oil until tender. Reduce heat to low.
7. On reduced heat, add the flour, sugar, molasses, mustard, vinegar, onion powder, and garlic.
8. Add the cooked beans, vegetable broth, and tomato paste.
9. Simmer for 15 minutes, stirring occasionally.
10. Add salt to taste.

Breakfast

(Pancakes, Waffles, French toast, Crepes, Potatoes, Muffins, Baked items, Hot cereal, and Miscellaneous)

Morning Pancakes

3 cups flour*
2 Tbs. sugar
1 Tbs. egg replacer powder
1 Tbs. baking powder
1½ tsp. baking soda

1 tsp. salt
3¼ cups soy milk
¼ cup extra light olive oil
2 Tbs. vanilla

*You can use half white flour and half whole wheat flour if you prefer.

* **Preheat griddle or skillet to 375°F, or choose the medium heat setting on your stove.**

1. In a large bowl, whisk together the flour, sugar, egg replacer, baking powder, baking soda, and salt.
2. Stir in the milk, oil, and vanilla.
3. Cook pancakes on a lightly oiled griddle, skillet or frying pan.

Variation: BRUNCH PANCAKES
In a blender, blend 6 oz. silken tofu with the milk, oil, and vanilla. Add blended ingredients to the dry ingredients.

Variation: FRUIT PANCAKES
Add 2 cups of fresh or thawed frozen fruit, such as blueberries, bananas, or apples.

Variation: HEALTHY PANCAKES
Reduce flour to 2¼ cups. Add ½ cup wheat or oat bran, ¼ cup ground flax seeds, and ¼ cup unsweetened protein powder.

Pumpkin Pancakes

Yield: 20 fat pancakes

1¼ cups whole wheat flour
1¼ cups white flour
3 Tbs. unsweetened brown rice or soy protein powder (optional)
¼ cup sugar
1½ Tbs. pumpkin pie spice
2 tsp. egg replacer powder

2 tsp. baking powder
2 tsp. baking soda
⅛ tsp. salt
2½ cups soy milk
2 Tbs. extra light olive oil
1 cup canned pumpkin

* Preheat griddle or skillet to 375°F, or choose the medium heat setting on your stove.

1. In a large bowl, whisk together the flours, protein powder, sugar, pumpkin pie spice, egg replacer, baking powder, baking soda, and salt.
2. Stir in the milk, oil, and pumpkin.
3. Cook pancakes on a lightly oiled griddle, skillet or frying pan.

Serve with applesauce or maple syrup.

Sourdough Pancakes

Yield: 36 4-inch pancakes

Sourdough starter:
1 Tbs. active dry yeast (¼-oz. package)
1 tsp. sugar
3 cups warm water (110°F)
3 cups flour

Pancake mix:
Sourdough starter

1 cup flour
1 cup soy milk
2 tsp. egg replacer powder
2 tsp. baking powder
1 tsp. salt
1 tsp. baking soda
¼ cup extra light olive oil
1 Tbs. vanilla

Sourdough starter:

1. In a large non-metal bowl, whisk together the yeast, sugar, and water. Let stand for 5 minutes.
2. Whisk in the 3 cups of flour. Cover with clear wrap and place in a warm (70–80°F) location for 12–24 hours. You may choose to keep the starter in your oven with the light turned on—just put a note on the stove to make sure you don't forget and turn on the oven. Stir starter once every 12 hours.

Pancakes:

1. Preheat electric griddle or skillet to 375°F, **or choose the medium heat setting on your stove.**
2. To your entire batch of sourdough starter (do not reserve any), whisk in all remaining ingredients.
3. Cook pancakes on a lightly oiled griddle, skillet or frying pan.

Variation: LEMON SOURDOUGH PANCAKES
Reduce soy milk to ¾ cup. Add zest of one lemon (minced) and juice of one lemon (¼ cup).

> **These are even more delicious when you warm up the maple syrup.**

Morning Waffles

Yield: 5 waffles

3 cups flour*
2 Tbs. baking powder
1 Tbs. egg replacer powder
1 tsp. salt
3 cups soy milk

⅓ cup extra light olive oil
1 tsp. vinegar
1 Tbs. vanilla
pan spray

*You can use half white flour and half whole wheat flour if you prefer.

*   Preheat waffle iron.

1. In a large bowl, whisk together the flour, baking powder, egg replacer and salt.
2. Whisk in the milk, oil, vinegar and vanilla.
3. Pan spray top and bottom of hot waffle iron if needed.
4. Scoop batter onto iron and cook for 4–5 minutes.

Variation: BRUNCH WAFFLES
Replace 2 cups of regular flour with 2 cups of semolina flour.

Variation: HEALTHY WAFFLES
Reduce flour to 2 cups. Add ½ cup of wheat or oat bran, ¼ cup ground flax seed, and ¼ cup unsweetened protein powder to the dry mix.

This version is good if you prefer a softer waffle. If you prefer a heartier waffle, try the Brunch Waffle variation.

French Toast

8 oz. silken tofu
1¼ cups soy milk
⅓ cup flour
3 Tbs. extra light olive oil
2 tsp. cinnamon
¾ tsp. baking powder

¾ tsp. egg replacer powder
½ tsp. salt
¼ tsp. nutmeg

16 slices of bread (sourdough or cinnamon swirl make it especially good!)

* Preheat griddle to 400°F, or choose the medium heat setting on your stove.

1. In a blender, blend tofu, soy milk, flour, oil, cinnamon, baking powder, egg replacer, salt, and nutmeg.
2. Pour batter into a shallow dish.
3. Lightly dip each side of the bread in the batter.
4. Cook on an oiled griddle or frying pan until browned on both sides.

Fresh sliced strawberries and pure maple syrup make an excellent French toast topping.

Blueberry Crepes

Yield: 16 crepes

2 cups flour
3 Tbs. sugar
2 Tbs. baking powder
1 tsp. salt
12⅓ oz. silken tofu (about 1½ cups)
3 cups soy milk

½ cup extra light olive oil
1 Tbs. vanilla
pan spray
blueberry sauce (p. 283), or one 21-oz. can
   prepared fruit topping

* Preheat griddle to 400°F, **or choose the medium heat setting on your stove.**

1. In a large bowl, whisk together flour, sugar, baking powder, and salt.
2. In a blender, blend tofu, soy milk, oil, and vanilla.
3. Whisk together the blended ingredients with the flour mixture.
4. Pan spray the griddle. Pour one quarter of the batter down the center of the griddle. Spread batter out evenly over the entire griddle.
5. When crepes are browned on the underside, make three cuts to divide crepes into 4 pieces. Flip crepes and cook for 2 more minutes. Roll crepes up and place on a cookie sheet in a 170° oven to keep warm while you finish the batch.
6. Top with blueberry sauce.

Variation: FRESH STRAWBERRY CREPES
Instead of prepared fruit topping, use 2 pints sliced fresh strawberries, with sweetener added as desired.

Crepes are quick and easy if you make 4 at a time, then top the finished crepes with fruit instead of filling and rolling them.

Hash Browns

4 medium potatoes, large dice (peeled if desired)
3 Tbs. light olive oil
salt to taste (about 1 tsp.)
pepper to taste (about ¼ tsp.)

* **Preheat oven to 475°F.**

1. Place potatoes in boiling water. Boil 10 minutes or until soft but not mushy.
2. Drain off water.
3. Toss potatoes with oil.
4. Place potatoes in a baking dish.
5. Bake, uncovered, for 20 minutes.
6. Add salt and pepper to taste.

Variation: COUNTRY-STYLE HASH BROWNS
While tossing the potatoes with the oil, add 1 diced bell pepper and ½ diced onion.

Variation: SEASONED HASH BROWNS
While tossing the potatoes with the oil, add 1 tsp. basil, paprika, garlic, and thyme.

Variation: SKILLET HASH BROWNS
After potatoes are boiled, place them in a large skillet with oil. Fry until browned. Add additional oil as needed.

Serve with country gravy (p. 280) if you like.

Potato Sausage Skillet

Yield: 4 servings

4 medium potatoes, ¾-inch dice (peeled if desired)

1 9-oz. package vegan breakfast sausages, thawed and chopped

½ onion, diced

1 bell pepper, diced

3 Tbs. light olive oil

¼ cup nutritional yeast flakes

½ tsp. garlic (optional)

salt to taste (about ¾ tsp.)

pepper to taste (about ¼ tsp.)

1. Place potatoes in boiling water. Boil 10 minutes or until soft but not mushy.
2. Drain off water.
3. In a large pan, sauté the sausage, onions, and pepper in the olive oil until onions are tender.
4. Add cooked potatoes, yeast flakes, and garlic. Continue to sauté for 3–5 minutes. Add additional oil as needed.
5. Add salt and pepper to taste.

Serve with country gravy (p. 280).

Banana Nut Muffins

Yield: 12 muffins

2½ cups flour*
½ cup sugar
1 Tbs. egg replacer powder
1 Tbs. baking powder
½ tsp. salt

2 ripe bananas, mashed
1¼ cups soy milk
⅓ cup extra light olive oil
2 tsp. vanilla
½ cup chopped walnuts

*You can use half white flour and half whole wheat flour if you prefer.

* **Preheat oven to 400°F.**

1. In a large bowl, whisk together the flour, sugar, egg replacer, baking powder, and salt.
2. With a spoon, stir in the bananas, milk, oil, vanilla, and nuts. Stir just until moistened.
3. Divide batter between 12 oiled muffin cups.
4. Bake for 20 minutes or until toothpick inserted in center comes out clean.

Variation: REDUCED-SUGAR BANANA NUT MUFFINS
Reduce sugar to ¼ cup and add ¼ tsp. powdered stevia extract.

Blueberry Muffins

Yield: 12 muffins

2½ cups flour*
½ cup sugar
1 Tbs. egg replacer powder
1 Tbs. baking powder
¾ tsp. salt

1½ cups soy milk
⅓ cup extra light olive oil
2 tsp. vanilla
1½ cups frozen blueberries**

*You can use half white flour and half whole wheat flour if you prefer.
**Preheat oven to only 400 degrees if using fresh or thawed blueberries.

*   Preheat oven to 425°F.

1. In a large bowl, whisk together the flour, sugar, egg replacer, baking powder, and salt.
2. With a spoon, stir in the milk, oil, vanilla, and blueberries. Stir just until moistened.
3. Divide batter between 12 oiled muffin cups.
4. Bake for 20 minutes or until toothpick inserted in center comes out clean.

Variation: REDUCED-SUGAR BLUEBERRY MUFFINS
Reduce sugar to ¼ cup and add ¼ tsp. powdered stevia extract.

Bake these muffins the night before to enjoy a stress-free breakfast.

Carrot Muffins

Yield: 12 muffins

2 cups flour*
¾ cup sugar
1 cup shredded carrot
¾ cup chopped walnuts
1 Tbs. egg replacer powder
1 Tbs. baking powder

1½ tsp. cinnamon
¼ tsp. nutmeg
¾ tsp. salt
1¼ cups soy milk
⅓ cup extra light olive oil
1 Tbs. vanilla

*You can use half white flour and half whole wheat flour if you prefer.

*   **Preheat oven to 400°F.**

1. In a large bowl, whisk together the flour, sugar, shredded carrots, walnuts, egg replacer, baking powder, cinnamon, nutmeg, and salt.
2. With a spoon, stir in the milk, oil, and vanilla. Stir just until moistened.
3. Divide batter between 12 oiled muffin cups.
4. Bake for 20 minutes or until toothpick inserted in center comes out clean.

Variation: REDUCED-SUGAR CARROT MUFFINS
Reduce sugar to ½ cup and add ¼ tsp. powdered stevia extract.

Good Morning Muffins

2 cups flour*
¾ cup sugar
½ cup oatmeal (uncooked)
1 Tbs. egg replacer powder
1 Tbs. baking powder
¾ tsp. salt

1 cup chopped walnuts
1½ cups soy milk
2 ripe bananas, mashed
⅓ cup extra light olive oil
2 tsp. maple extract
1 Tbs. vanilla

*You can use half white flour and half whole wheat flour if you prefer.

* **Preheat oven to 400°F.**

1. In a large bowl, whisk together the flour, sugar, oatmeal, egg replacer, baking powder, and salt.
2. With a spoon, stir in the walnuts, soy milk, bananas, oil, maple extract, and vanilla. Stir just until moistened.
3. Divide batter between 16 oiled muffin cups.
4. Bake for 20 minutes or until toothpick inserted in center comes out clean.

Variation: REDUCED-SUGAR GOOD MORNING MUFFINS
Reduce sugar to ⅓ cup and add ½ tsp. powdered stevia extract.

A maple and banana muffin with oatmeal and walnuts.

Lemon Poppy Seed Muffins

Yield: 12 muffins

2½ cups flour*
¾ cup sugar
⅓ cup poppy seeds
1 Tbs. egg replacer powder
1 Tbs. baking powder
½ tsp. salt

1¼ cups soy milk
⅓ cup extra light olive oil
2 tsp. vanilla
zest of 2 lemons, minced (2 Tbs.)
juice of 2 lemons (½ cup)

*You can use half white flour and half whole wheat flour if you prefer.

---

*   **Preheat oven to 400°F.**

1.   In a large bowl, whisk together the flour, sugar, poppy seeds, egg replacer, baking powder, and salt.
2.   With a spoon, stir in the soy milk, olive oil, vanilla, lemon zest, and lemon juice. Stir just until moistened.
3.   Divide batter between 12 oiled muffin cups.
4.   Bake for 18 minutes or until toothpick inserted in center comes out clean.

Variation: REDUCED-SUGAR LEMON POPPY SEED MUFFINS
Reduce sugar to ½ cup and add ¼ tsp. powdered stevia extract.

Maple Pecan & Date Muffins

Yield: 12 muffins

2½ cups flour*
½ cup sugar
1 Tbs. egg replacer powder
1 Tbs. baking powder
¾ tsp. salt
¾ cup chopped dates

¾ cup maple chunks**
¾ cup chopped pecans
1½ cups soy milk
⅓ cup extra light olive oil
2 tsp. maple extract

*You can use half white flour and half whole wheat flour if you prefer.
**Maple chunks can usually be found in the baking aisle in natural food stores.

*   **Preheat oven to 400°F.**

1. In a large bowl, whisk together the flour, sugar, egg replacer, baking powder, and salt.
2. With a spoon, stir in the dates, maple chunks, pecans, soy milk, oil, and maple extract.
3. Divide batter between 12 oiled muffin cups.
4. Bake for 20 minutes or until toothpick inserted in center comes out clean.

Variation: REDUCED-SUGAR MAPLE PECAN AND DATE MUFFINS
Reduce sugar to ¼ cup and add ¼ tsp. powdered stevia extract. Reduce chopped dates and maple chunks to ⅓ cup each.

Oat Bran Muffins

Yield: 12 muffins

1 cup white flour
1 cup whole wheat flour
1 cup oat bran
½ cup + 2 Tbs. sugar
¼ cup ground flax seeds (optional)
1 Tbs. egg replacer powder

1 Tbs. baking powder
1 tsp. salt
1½ cups soy milk
⅓ cup extra light olive oil
1 Tbs. vanilla

* Preheat oven to 400°F.

1. In a large bowl, whisk together the flours, bran, sugar, flax seed, egg replacer, baking powder, and salt.
2. With a spoon, stir in the milk, oil, and vanilla, just until moistened.
3. Divide batter between 12 oiled muffin cups.
4. Bake for 18 minutes or until toothpick inserted in center comes out clean.

Variation: RAISIN NUT OAT BRAN MUFFINS
Add ¾ cup raisins and ¾ cup chopped walnuts. Increase baking time to 20 minutes.

Variation: CARROT OAT BRAN MUFFINS
Add 2 cups shredded carrots, 1½ tsp. cinnamon, and ¼ tsp. nutmeg. Increase baking time to 20 minutes.

Variation: REDUCED-SUGAR OAT BRAN MUFFINS
Reduce sugar to ¼ cup and add ¼ tsp. powdered stevia extract.

Pumpkin Muffins

Yield: 12 muffins

2½ cups flour*
¾ cup sugar
1 Tbs. egg replacer powder
1 Tbs. baking powder
2 tsp. cinnamon
¾ tsp. salt

¼ tsp. nutmeg
1¼ cups soy milk
1 cup canned pumpkin
⅓ cup extra light olive oil
2 Tbs. molasses
1 tsp. vanilla

*You can use half white flour and half whole wheat flour if you prefer.

---

*   **Preheat oven to 400°F.**

1. In a large bowl, whisk together the flour, sugar, egg replacer, baking powder, cinnamon, salt, and nutmeg.
2. With a spoon, stir in the soy milk, pumpkin, oil, molasses, and vanilla. Stir just until moistened.
3. Divide batter between 12 oiled muffin cups.
4. Bake for 20 minutes or until toothpick inserted in center comes out clean.

Variation: RAISIN WALNUT PUMPKIN MUFFINS
Add ¾ cup raisins and ¾ cup chopped walnuts.

Variation: REDUCED-SUGAR PUMPKIN MUFFINS
Reduce sugar to ½ cup and add ¼ tsp. powdered stevia extract.

Wheat Bran Muffins

Yield: 12 muffins

---

1 cup white flour	1 Tbs. baking powder
1 cup whole wheat flour	1 tsp. salt
1 cup wheat bran	1½ cups soy milk
½ cup sugar	⅓ cup extra light olive oil
¼ cup ground flax seeds (optional)	3 Tbs. molasses
1 Tbs. egg replacer powder	1 Tbs. vanilla

---

*   **Preheat oven to 400°F.**

1. In a large bowl, whisk together the flours, bran, sugar, flax seeds, egg replacer, baking powder, and salt.
2. With a spoon, stir in the soy milk, oil, molasses, and vanilla. Stir just until moistened.
3. Divide batter between 12 oiled muffin cups.
4. Bake for 18 minutes or until toothpick inserted in center comes out clean.

Variation: RAISIN NUT WHEAT BRAN MUFFINS

Add ¾ cup raisins and ¾ cup chopped walnuts. Increase baking time to 20 minutes.

Variation: CARROT WHEAT BRAN MUFFINS

Add 2 cups shredded carrots, 1½ tsp. cinnamon, and ¼ tsp. nutmeg. Increase baking time to 20 minutes.

Variation: REDUCED-SUGAR WHEAT BRAN MUFFINS

Reduce sugar to ¼ cup and add ¼ tsp. powdered stevia extract.

Drop Biscuits

3½ cups flour*
5 tsp. baking powder
1½ tsp. salt
1½ cups soy milk
⅗ cup extra light olive oil

*You can use half white flour and half whole wheat flour if you prefer.

---

*   **Preheat oven to 450°F.**

1.   In a large bowl, whisk together the flour, baking powder, and salt.
2.   With a spoon, stir in the soy milk and oil. Stir just until moistened.
3.   Scoop or spoon biscuits onto a lightly oiled cookie sheet.
4.   Bake for 12 minutes or until toothpick inserted in center comes out clean.

Variation: CUTOUT BISCUITS
Increase flour to 4 cups. On a floured surface, roll out dough to 1 inch thick. Using your favorite cookie cutter, cut out biscuits and place on a lightly oiled cookie sheet.

Variation: ITALIAN HERB BISCUITS
Add 2 tsp. basil, 1 tsp. oregano to flour mixture.

Variation: TRADITIONAL HERB BISCUITS
Add 1 Tbs. parsley flakes, 1 tsp. thyme, and ½ tsp. sage to flour mixture.

Cinnamon Roll Biscuits

Yield: 8 biscuits

Cutout biscuit dough (p. 131)
1 Tbs. cinnamon
¾ cup brown sugar
¼ cup melted margarine or ¼ cup extra
    light olive oil

*   **Preheat oven to 425°F.**

1. Prepare dough according to the cutout biscuit recipe.
2. On a floured surface, roll out dough to 12 x 16 inches.
3. Pour melted margarine or oil on dough and spread out evenly. Sprinkle with cinnamon and brown sugar.
4. Roll dough into a 12-inch roll.
5. Cut into 8 rolls of equal size. Place in an oiled 9 x 13-inch baking dish.
6. Bake for 18 minutes or until toothpick inserted in the center comes out clean.

Coffee Cake

Yield: 12 pieces

3 cups flour*
1 cup sugar
1 tsp. cinnamon
½ tsp. nutmeg
½ tsp. allspice

½ tsp. salt
¾ cup extra light olive oil
1 Tbs. baking powder
1 cup soy milk

*You can use half white flour and half whole wheat flour if you prefer.

* **Preheat oven to 375°F.**

1. In a large bowl, whisk together the flour, sugar, cinnamon, nutmeg, allspice, and salt.
2. With a fork, cut in the oil until mixture looks like a crumb topping.
3. Reserve 1½ cups of this mixture for the topping.
4. Add soy milk and baking powder to the non-reserved mix to make the batter. Mix well.
5. Spread batter in an oiled 9 x 13-inch baking dish.
6. Sprinkle the 1½ cups reserved topping on top of batter.
7. Bake for 25 minutes or until toothpick inserted in center comes out clean.

Variation: APPLE WALNUT COFFEE CAKE

Combine 2 small apples (peeled, cored, and small dice) and 1 cup chopped walnuts to the reserved crumb topping before sprinkling on top of batter. Increase cooking time to 30 minutes.

Variation: REDUCED-SUGAR COFFEE CAKE

Reduce sugar to ½ cup and add ½ tsp. powdered stevia extract.

> **If you are having guests over, try the Apple Walnut Coffee Cake.**

Scones

2½ cups flour*
⅓ cup sugar
2 tsp. baking powder
½ tsp. baking soda
½ tsp. salt
½ cup currants or raisins (optional)
⅓ cup margarine

6 oz. silken tofu
¾ cup soy milk
1 tsp. vinegar
2 tsp. vanilla
½ tsp. almond extract
1 Tbs. sugar

*You can use half white flour and half whole wheat flour if you prefer.

* **Preheat oven to 425°F.**

1. In large bowl, whisk together the flour, ⅓ cup sugar, baking powder, baking soda, salt, and currants.
2. In a blender, blend the margarine, tofu, soy milk, vinegar, vanilla, and almond extract.
3. Spoon blended ingredients into flour mixture. Stir until just moistened.
4. Scoop 12 individual scones onto an oiled cookie sheet and flatten slightly.
5. Sprinkle the 1 Tbs. sugar on top of slightly flattened scones.
6. Bake for 17 minutes or until toothpick inserted in center comes out clean.

Variation: HOLIDAY SCONES
Substitute dried cranberries for the currants and add 1 tsp. pumpkin pie spice.

Variation: WALNUT SCONES
Add ¾ cup chopped walnuts.

Hot Breakfast Cereals

Yield: 4–5 servings

FARINA

4 cups soy milk
1½ cups non-instant farina

Heat soy milk to a near boil. Reduce heat to low. Slowly stir in farina with whisk and stir well for 2 minutes. Cook for 8 more minutes, stirring frequently.

KAMUT

4 cups soy milk
2 cups kamut

Heat soy milk to a near boil. Reduce heat to low. Stir in kamut and stir well for the first minute. Cook for 9 more minutes, stirring frequently.

OATMEAL

4 cups soy milk
2 cups quick oats

Bring soy milk to a near boil. Reduce heat to low. Stir in oats and continue to stir for one minute. Cook for about 4 more minutes, stirring frequently.

POLENTA

4 cups soy milk
1¼ cups polenta
2 Tbs. margarine (optional)

Bring soy milk to a near boil. Reduce heat to low. Stir in polenta. Continue to cook for 20 minutes, stirring frequently. Stir in margarine.

> **As a topping, try dried fruit, fresh fruit, applesauce, maple syrup, granola, chopped nuts, stevia, coconut, molasses, date sugar, cinnamon, or nutmeg.**

Fruit & Yogurt Cup

6 oz. fruit soy yogurt
1 cup fresh fruit (sliced strawberries, blueberries, etc.)
¼ cup granola

1. In a parfait cup, layer a third of the yogurt, half the granola, and half the fresh fruit, repeat.
2. Place last third of yogurt on top.

"Maple" Syrup

Yield: 2 cups

1 cup sugar
1 cup brown sugar
1 cup water
2 tsp. maple extract

1. In a saucepan, combine all ingredients.
2. Bring to a boil, reduce heat to low, and simmer for 5 minutes. Watch carefully, because it tends to boil over.
3. Store leftovers in refrigerator.

A homemade substitute
for maple syrup.

Lunch

(Sandwiches, Wraps, Entrées)

Sandwiches

Wraps

Entrées

Grilled "Cheese" Sandwich

Yield: 5 sandwiches

1¼ cups soy milk
⅓ cup uncooked oatmeal
⅓ cup peanut, almond, or soy butter
⅓ cup nutritional yeast flakes
1 2-oz. jar pimientos
2 Tbs. cornstarch

2 Tbs. lemon juice
1½ tsp. salt
¼ tsp. paprika
pinch of cayenne (optional)
10 slices bread

*   Preheat griddle or skillet to 375°F, or choose the medium heat setting on your stove.

1. In a blender, blend the soy milk, oatmeal, nut butter, yeast flakes, pimientos, cornstarch, lemon juice, salt, paprika, and cayenne until smooth.
2. Pour into saucepan and cook until thickened, stirring constantly.
3. Spread "cheese" between slices of bread.
4. Grill sandwiches on a lightly oiled griddle until browned on each side.

Add some vegan pepperoni to your sandwich for a treat.

Grilled Eggplant Sandwich

Yield: 3 sandwiches

1 eggplant
2 Tbs. light olive oil
½ tsp. salt
½ tsp. garlic (optional)
¼ tsp. basil
¼ tsp. thyme

6 slices vegan cheese
6 slices bread (preferably sourdough)

* Preheat griddle to 375°F, or choose the medium heat setting on your stove.

1. Peel eggplant and cut into ½-inch slabs.
2. In a small bowl, combine oil, salt, garlic, basil, and thyme.
3. Brush both sides of eggplant with oil mixture.
4. Grill eggplant for 4 minutes on each side.
5. Place grilled eggplant and cheese between two slices of bread.
6. Place sandwiches on oiled griddle and brown on each side.

Variation: GRILLED EGGPLANT SANDWICH WITH ROASTED VEGETABLES
Add ¼ cup roasted vegetables (p. 71) per sandwich before grilling.

Grilled Portobello Sandwich

Yield: 2 sandwiches

---

2 large portobello mushrooms
2 Tbs. light olive oil
½ tsp. salt
½ tsp. garlic (optional)
¼ tsp. basil
¼ tsp. thyme

4 slices vegan cheese
4 slices bread (preferably sourdough)

---

*   **Preheat griddle to 375°F, or choose the medium heat setting on your stove.**

1.   Remove stems from mushrooms and discard. Lightly rinse and pat dry.
2.   In a small bowl, combine oil, salt, garlic, basil, and thyme.
3.   Brush both sides of portobellos with oil mixture.
4.   Grill portobellos for 4 minutes on each side or until soft.
5.   Place grilled mushrooms and cheese between two slices of bread.
6.   Place sandwiches on oiled griddle and brown on each side.

Variation: GRILLED PORTOBELLO SANDWICH WITH CARAMELIZED ONION AND GARLIC SPREAD
Spread 1 or 2 Tbs. caramelized onion and garlic spread (p. 290) inside the bread before grilling.

Vegetable Burger

2 cups oatmeal (uncooked)
½ cup wheat gluten
½ cup nutritional yeast flakes
1 carrot, shredded
1 small zucchini, shredded
½ onion, diced
1 shallot, minced
4 cloves garlic, minced (optional)

½ cup frozen shelled soybeans (thawed)
½ cup corn
1 2-oz. jar pimientos
¼ cup light olive oil
2 Tbs. soy sauce*
salt to taste (about 1¾ tsp.)

*Substitute Bragg liquid aminos if you prefer.

* **Preheat griddle to 400°F, or choose the medium heat setting on your stove.**

1. In a large bowl, mix all ingredients except salt.
2. Place ¾ of the mixture into a food processor. Process until well mixed.
3. Add processed mixture back into the large bowl with the remaining mixture and stir.
4. Add salt to taste.
5. Form 12 patties.
6. Grill on lightly oiled griddle until browned on both sides.

Makes a great side dish or entrée.

Rainbow Wrap

6 large flour tortillas
¼ small head red cabbage, shredded
¼ bunch spinach, chopped
1 yam, shredded
1 zucchini, shredded
1 cup hummus (p. 11)

1. Soften tortillas for easier rolling by warming them in a microwave, grill top, or oven.
2. Place ⅙ of the ingredients in each tortilla.
3. Roll up burrito-style.

Eating a mixture of different-colored raw vegetables is a good way to provide a variety of vitamins in your diet.

Roasted Vegetable Wrap

Yield: 6 wraps

6 large flour tortillas
3 cups roasted vegetables (p. 71)
3 cups shredded lettuce
6 tomato slices
1 cup hummus (p. 11)

1. Soften tortillas for easier rolling by warming them in a microwave, grill top, or oven.
2. Place ⅙ of the ingredients in each tortilla.
3. Roll up burrito-style.

Substitute roasted vegetable "cream cheese" spread (p. 292) for the hummus if you'd like.

Thai Wrap

Yield: 6 wraps

6 large flour tortillas
3 cups cooked jasmine rice (p. 96)
¼ head red cabbage, shredded
3 carrots, shredded
1 head iceberg lettuce, shredded
1 pound bean sprouts, well rinsed

1 bunch cilantro, chopped
1 bunch green onions, chopped
1 cup peanut sauce (p. 285)

1. Soften tortillas for easier rolling by warming them in a microwave, grill top, or oven.
2. Place ⅙ of the ingredients in each tortilla.
3. Roll up burrito-style.

Baked Potato Bar

6 large potatoes
1 Tbs. light olive oil

*   **Preheat oven to 425°F.**

1. Wash potatoes.
2. Jab each potato a few times with a fork.
3. Lightly oil each potato.
4. Bake 1 to 1½ hours or until soft.
5. While potatoes are cooking, prep desired toppings and place in individual bowls.

Topping Suggestions:

Chili, heated
Margarine
Light olive oil
Vegan cheese sauce
Shredded vegan cheese
Broccoli, bite-sized (raw or steamed)
Green onions, chopped
Onion, chopped (raw or sautéed)
Mushrooms, sliced (raw or sautéed)
Black olives
Sunflower seeds
Tomatoes, diced
Canned jalapeños, sliced
Salsa
Nutritional yeast flakes
Salt
Pepper

BBQ Green Chili Pizza

Yield: 14-inch pizza

Pizza crust, uncooked (p. 209)
Pizza sauce (p. 287)
5 oz. vegan BBQ riblets, thawed & diced
1 4-oz. can diced green chilies
½ onion, diced
10 oz. shredded vegan mozzarella or Monterey jack cheese

1. Roll out pizza dough on oiled cookie sheet.
2. Cover dough with pizza sauce, 4 oz. of cheese, BBQ riblets, green chilies, and onion.
3. Top with remaining cheese.
4. Let rest on counter for 30 minutes to allow dough to rise.
5. Preheat oven to 450°F.
6. Bake pizza for 15 minutes or until done.

Beanie Weenies

Yield: 6 servings

2 15-oz. cans vegan baked beans
8 vegan hot dogs, sliced

1. In a 3-quart saucepan, combine beans and hot dogs.
2. Heat and serve.

For when you need a very
quick meal.

Chow Mein

3 7-oz. packages fresh soba noodles*
¼ cup sesame oil
3 ribs celery, diced
½ onion, diced
1 bell pepper, julienne cut
2 carrots, julienne cut

4 mushrooms, sliced
1 Tbs. fresh ginger, minced
1 5-oz. can water chestnuts (drained)
1 5-oz. can bamboo shoots (drained)
soy sauce** to taste (about ⅓ cup)

*Usually sold in the produce section of the supermarket. You can substitute 12 oz. cooked spaghetti if you prefer.
**Substitute Bragg liquid aminos if you prefer.

1. Boil soba noodles for 3 minutes. Drain off water and set noodles aside.
2. In a large pan, sauté the celery, onion, pepper, carrots, mushrooms, and ginger with the sesame oil until tender, but still crisp.
3. Add noodles, water chestnuts, and bamboo shoots. Continue to sauté until all ingredients are hot.
4. Add soy sauce to taste.

This is a versatile recipe that you can add to or subtract from as you like.

Macaroni & "Cheese"

Yield: 6 servings

16 oz. uncooked macaroni noodles
2¼ cups soy milk
½ cup nutritional yeast flakes
¼ cup flour
¼ cup light olive oil
1 2-oz. jar diced pimientos

2 Tbs. peanut, almond, or soy butter
1 tsp. onion powder
¾ tsp. paprika
salt to taste (about 1¾ tsp.)

1. Cook pasta according to package directions. Drain and set aside.
2. In a blender, blend soy milk, yeast flakes, flour, oil, pimientos, nut butter, onion powder, and paprika.
3. Pour into a 2-quart saucepan and cook over medium heat until hot and thickened, stirring frequently.
4. Add salt to taste.
5. Mix cheese sauce with the cooked macaroni.

Variation: ITALIAN-STYLE MACARONI & "CHEESE"
Add ¼ cup Italian dressing (p. 60) while blending. Add ½ cup sliced black olives to the cheese sauce while it is cooking.

Variation: MEXICAN-STYLE MACARONI & "CHEESE"
Add one 4-oz. can diced green chilies and ¼ tsp. chili powder to the cheese sauce while it is cooking.

Nachos

2 cups soy milk
2 Tbs. light olive oil
¼ cup flour
1 4-oz. can diced green chilies
1 2-oz. jar pimientos
½ cup nutritional yeast flakes

2 Tbs. peanut, almond, or soy butter
1 tsp. garlic
½ tsp. chili powder
salt to taste (about 1¾ tsp.)
1 16-oz. bag tortilla chips

1. In a blender, blend the soy milk, oil, flour, pimientos, green chilies, yeast flakes, almond butter, garlic, and chili powder.
2. Pour sauce into a 2-quart saucepan and cook until hot and thickened, stirring constantly.
3. Add salt to taste.
4. Pour sauce over chips and add toppings of your choice.

Optional toppings:
Soy taco filling, heated
Refried beans, heated
Diced tomatoes
Sliced black olives
Chopped green onions
Salsa
Guacamole

Try warming the chips in a 170° oven for a couple of minutes before serving.

Weiner Wraps

Yield: 8 wraps

Cutout biscuit dough (p. 131)
8 vegan hot dogs

*   **Preheat oven to 450°F.**

1. Prepare dough according to the cutout biscuit recipe.
2. On a floured surface, roll out dough to 12 x 16 inches.
3. Cut into 8 rectangular pieces, 4 x 3 inches each.
4. Wrap one piece of dough around each veggie dog.
5. Place on oiled cookie sheet.

Bake for 15 minutes or until toothpick inserted in middle of dough comes out clean.

> **This quick meal is an easy way to serve up lunch or dinner in a snap. Don't forget the mustard.**

Dinner

(American, Mediterranean, Thai, Indian, Asian, Mexican)

Biscuit Casserole Stew

Yield: 8 servings

Drop biscuit dough (p. 131)
2 potatoes, diced
¼ cup light olive oil
1 carrot, diced
3 ribs celery, diced
1 onion, diced
⅓ cup flour

1 tsp. garlic (optional)
1 tsp. thyme
1 12-oz. can ready-to-serve split pea soup
4 cups vegetable broth
salt to taste (about 1½ tsp.)
black pepper to taste (about ¼ tsp.)

* **Preheat oven to 400°F.**

1. Boil potatoes for 10 minutes. Drain off water and set potatoes aside.
2. In a large saucepan, sauté the carrot, celery, and onion in the oil until vegetables are tender. Reduce heat to low.
3. On reduced heat, add flour, garlic, and thyme. Sauté for 2 minutes.
4. Stir in split pea soup, potatoes, and vegetable broth. Bring stew to a boil, reduce heat to low, and simmer for 10 minutes, stirring frequently. Add salt and pepper to taste.
5. While stew is simmering, prepare biscuit dough.
6. Pour stew into a 10 x 15-inch baking dish.
7. Drop 15 uncooked biscuit dough balls on top of the stew.
8. Bake, uncovered, for 20 minutes or until toothpick inserted in middle of biscuit comes out clean.

Davis Apple Stew

Yield: 5 servings

¼ cup light olive oil
1 potato, diced
½ onion, diced
1 sweet potato, diced
2 carrots, diced
2 green apples, peeled, cored, and diced

⅓ cup flour
1 tsp. thyme
1 tsp. garlic (optional)
3 cups vegetable broth
salt to taste (about 1½ tsp.)
pepper to taste (about ¼ tsp.)

1. In a large pot, sauté the potato, onion, sweet potato, and carrots in the oil until tender. Reduce heat to low.
2. On reduced heat, add the apples, flour, thyme, and garlic. Continue to sauté for 2 more minutes.
3. Add the vegetable broth. Turn up heat and cook until hot and thickened.
4. Simmer for 5 minutes.
5. Add salt and pepper to taste.

Fennel Root Stew

1 fennel root, peeled and diced
3 carrots, diced
3 ribs celery, diced
½ onion, diced
¼ cup light olive oil
8 mushrooms, sliced

⅓ cup flour
1 tsp. garlic (optional)
¼ tsp. ground black pepper
2 cups prepared vegetable broth
2 cups prepared mushroom soup
salt to taste (about 1½ tsp.)

1. In a large saucepan, sauté the fennel, carrots, celery, and onion in the oil until vegetables are tender. Reduce heat to low.
2. On reduced heat, add mushrooms, flour, garlic, and black pepper. Sauté for 3 more minutes.
3. Turn up heat to medium. Add the vegetable broth and mushroom soup. Heat stew until hot and thickened, stirring frequently.
4. Add salt to taste.

Serve with rustic bread.

Mushroom & Wild Rice Crepes

Yield: 16 crepes (4 servings)

Mushroom and wild rice (p. 98)
16 crepes (p. 296)

1. Prepare mushroom and wild rice according to the directions on p. 98.
2. Prepare crepes according to the directions on p. 296.
3. Fill crepes with rice mixture and roll up.

A nice dish for a quiet evening meal.

Pasta Bake with Vegetables

8 oz. uncooked penne pasta
2 cups bite-sized broccoli pieces
2 cups bite-sized cauliflower pieces
3 cups soy milk
⅓ cup flour
¼ cup nutritional yeast flakes

⅛ tsp. nutmeg
¼ cup light olive oil
salt to taste (about 1¼ tsp.)
¼ cup vegan parmesan cheese (p. 298)
½ cup slivered almonds

* **Preheat oven to 400°F.**

1. Cook pasta according to package directions. Drain off water and set pasta aside.
2. Place broccoli and cauliflower in boiling water and boil for 3 minutes. Drain off water and set vegetables aside.
3. In a blender, blend the soy milk, flour, yeast flakes, nutmeg, and oil until smooth.
4. Pour blended ingredients into a 3-quart saucepan. Heat sauce until hot and thickened, stirring frequently.
5. Add salt to taste.
6. In a 9 x 13-inch baking dish, combine the pasta, broccoli, cauliflower, and sauce. Top with parmesan cheese and almonds.
7. Bake, uncovered, for 10 minutes.

Pasta with Pepper Cream Sauce

Yield: 3 servings

8 oz. uncooked pasta
1 green bell pepper, julienne cut
1 red bell pepper, julienne cut
½ onions, julienne cut
1 6-oz. package seasoned vegetarian
    chicken strips

¼ cup light olive oil
¼ cup flour
2 cups soy milk
salt to taste (about 1 tsp.)
pepper to taste (about ½ tsp.)

1. Cook pasta according to package directions.
2. In a large pot, sauté the peppers, onion, and veggie strips in the oil until vegetables are tender. Reduce heat to low.
3. On reduced heat, add flour. Sauté for 1 minute.
4. Add soy milk. Turn up heat to medium and cook until hot and thickened, stirring frequently.
5. Add salt and pepper to taste.
6. Combine with cooked pasta.

Red Beans & Rice

Yield: 5 servings

1 carrot, diced
1 small onion, diced
2 Tbs. light olive oil
¾ tsp. sage
¾ tsp. marjoram
½ cup dry adzuki beans

2½ cups vegetable broth
¾ cup brown rice, rinsed
1½ cups vegetable broth
¼ cup water
salt to taste (about 1 tsp.)
2 tomatoes, diced

1. In a large pan, sauté the carrot and onion in the oil until tender. Add marjoram and sage. Sauté 1 more minute.
2. Add beans and vegetable broth. Bring to a boil, reduce heat to low, cover, and simmer for 1½ to 2 hours or until beans are tender, stirring occasionally.
3. In a 2-quart saucepan, add rice, 1½ cups vegetable broth, and water. Bring to a boil, reduce heat to low, cover, and simmer for 45 minutes.
4. Add cooked rice to cooked beans.
5. Add salt to taste.
6. Add tomatoes right before serving.

Vegan Turkey

1 gallon water
2½ cups vital wheat gluten flour
½ cup nutritional yeast flakes
1 tsp. thyme
1 Tbs. onion powder
1 tsp. salt

2 cups vegetable broth*
¼ cup light olive oil
1 Tbs. soy sauce**
cheesecloth (one double-thick 24 x 16-inch piece)
2 6-inch pieces of string

*If using the homemade vegetable broth on p. 300, you may need to add salt to this recipe.
**Substitute Bragg liquid aminos if desired.

1. In a large pot, bring 1 gallon of water to a simmer.
2. In a large bowl, whisk together the gluten, yeast flakes, thyme, onion powder, and salt.
3. Add the vegetable broth, oil, and soy sauce, and stir just until combined.
4. Form into a loaf shape.
5. Place gluten loaf on cheesecloth and roll up (not too tight). Tie each end with a piece of string.
6. Place in simmering water, covered, for 1 hour.***
7. Preheat oven to 325°F.
8. Take roast out of water and remove cheesecloth. Place in baking dish.
9. Bake, covered, for 30 minutes.

***Make stuffing (see Side Dishes, p. 88) while turkey is simmering in the water. Cook the stuffing in the baking dish with the turkey.

Also makes great sandwiches!

Vegetable Noodle Casserole

8 oz. uncooked curly noodles
½ onion, diced
3 ribs celery, diced
2 carrots, diced
¼ cup light olive oil
⅓ cup flour

2 cups soy milk
2 cups vegetable broth
salt to taste (about 1½ tsp.)
1½ cups shredded vegan cheddar cheese
1 cup crushed potato chips (5-oz. bag)

*   **Preheat oven to 400°F.**

1. Cook pasta according to packaged directions.
2. Place cooked pasta in a 9 x 13-inch baking dish.
3. In a 3-quart saucepan, sauté the onion, celery, and carrots in the oil until tender. Reduce heat to low.
4. On reduced heat, add flour and sauté for 2 minutes, stirring often.
5. Add the soy milk and vegetable broth and increase heat to medium/high. Cook until thickened, stirring frequently.
6. Add salt to taste.
7. Combine sauce and pasta in the baking dish.
8. Top with cheese and potato chips.
9. Bake, uncovered, for 10 minutes.

> **For a cheesier flavor, add 1/4 cup nutritional yeast flakes to the sauce.**

Vegetable Quiche Pie

Yield: One 9-inch pie

1 9-inch single uncooked pie crust (p. 233)
2 Tbs. light olive oil
1 small sweet onion, diced
2 carrots, diced
4 ribs celery, diced
1 cup firm or extra firm tofu

¼ cup nutritional yeast flakes
3 Tbs. cornstarch
1 Tbs. flour
1½ tsp. salt
⅛ tsp. black pepper
⅛ tsp. nutmeg

* **Preheat oven to 350°F.**

1. Prepare pie crust and place in a 9-inch round pie dish. Cover and set aside.
2. Sauté onions, carrots, and celery with oil until tender.
3. In a food processor, mix the tofu, yeast flakes, cornstarch, flour, salt, pepper, and nutmeg until smooth. Transfer to a large bowl.
4. Add sautéed vegetables.
5. Transfer to prepared pie crust.
6. Bake, uncovered, for 45 minutes.

Vegetable Scrambler

½ onion, diced
8 mushrooms, sliced
2 Tbs. light olive oil
1 pound firm tofu, crumbled
1 tomato, diced
½ bunch spinach, chopped

¾ tsp. garlic (optional)
½ tsp. thyme
½ tsp. turmeric
salt to taste (about ¾ tsp.)

1. In a large pan, sauté the onions and mushrooms in the oil until tender.
2. Add tofu, tomato, spinach, garlic, thyme, and turmeric. Sauté for 5 more minutes.
3. Add salt to taste.

Serve with warm corn bread or toast.

Fresh Herb & Garlic Pasta

16 oz. uncooked pasta
1 cup sun-dried tomatoes
¼ cup fresh garlic, peeled and chopped
1 bunch fresh basil, stemmed and chopped
1 bunch fresh oregano, stemmed and
   chopped

1 small sweet white onion, diced
1 green bell pepper, diced
1 red bell pepper, diced
½ cup light olive oil
salt to taste (about 2 tsp.)

1. Cook pasta according to package directions.
2. Boil sun-dried tomatoes for 5 minutes. Drain off water. (Omit this step if using sun-dried tomatoes that come packed in oil.)
3. In a food processor, add sun-dried tomatoes, garlic, basil, oregano, onion, peppers, and oil. Process well.
4. Pour sauce into large pan and sauté for 5 minutes. Add salt to taste.
5. Toss with hot pasta and serve.

This gourmet, flavor-intense cuisine will delight your guests.

Lasagna Florentine

Yield: 6 servings

8 oz. uncooked lasagna noodles
¼ cup + 1 Tbs. light olive oil
1 bell pepper, diced
½ onion, diced
2 tsp. basil
1 tsp. garlic

1 tsp. onion powder
½ cup flour
1 tsp. salt
1 bunch spinach, chopped
⅓ cup vegan parmesan cheese (p. 298)
3 cups soy milk

*   Preheat oven to 375°F.

1. Boil lasagna noodles just until soft. Drain off water and cool down noodles with cold water. Place noodles in a bowl and toss with 1 Tbs. oil.
2. In a 3-quart saucepan, sauté pepper and onion in ¼ cup oil until tender. Reduce heat to low.
3. On reduced heat, add basil, garlic, onion powder, flour, and salt. Sauté for 2 minutes. Add spinach and sauté until wilted.
4. Add soy milk and parmesan cheese. Turn up heat to medium and cook until sauce is thickened.
5. In an 8 x 8-inch baking dish, layer 5 layers of sauce and 4 layers of noodles, starting and ending with the sauce.
6. Bake, covered, for 25 minutes. Remove from oven and cool for 10 minutes before serving.

Moroccan Black Bean Stew

Yield: 6 servings

4 cups prepared couscous (p. 107)
½ onion, diced
1 small yam, peeled and diced
1 small zucchini, diced
1 red bell pepper, diced
¼ cup light olive oil
3 Tbs. flour
2 Tbs. sugar

2 tsp. curry powder
1 tsp. cinnamon
2 cups vegetable broth
1 15-oz. can black beans, drained and
   rinsed
½ cup raisins
salt to taste (about 1½ tsp.)

1. In a large pot, sauté the onion, yam, zucchini, and pepper in the oil until vegetables are tender. Reduce heat to low.
2. On reduced heat, add the flour, sugar, curry, and cinnamon. Sauté for 1 minute.
3. Add the vegetable broth, black beans, and raisins. Turn up heat and cook stew until hot and thickened.
4. Add salt to taste.
5. Serve on a bed of couscous.

An exotic dish with many flavors and colors.

Pasta with Marinara Sauce

Yield: 5 servings

16 oz. uncooked pasta
½ onion, diced
3 Tbs. light olive oil
1 Tbs. basil
2 tsp. onion powder (optional)
2 tsp. oregano

1 tsp. sugar
1 28-oz. can crushed or diced tomatoes
1 6-oz. can tomato paste
salt to taste (about 2 tsp.)

1. Cook pasta according to package directions.
2. In a 3-quart saucepan, sauté the onion in the oil until tender. Reduce heat to low.
3. On reduced heat, add the basil, onion powder, oregano, and sugar. Sauté for 1 minute.
4. Add tomatoes and tomato paste.
5. Cover and simmer for 15 minutes, stirring occasionally.
6. Add salt to taste.

Serve with an herb baguette (p. 4) and crisp Caesar salad (p. 35).

Pesto Pasta

Yield: 6 servings

16 oz. uncooked pasta
2 bunches fresh basil, stemmed and
    chopped
⅓ cup light olive oil
1 head of fresh garlic, peeled (about 16
    cloves)

½ cup pine nuts
salt to taste (about 1½ tsp.)

1. Cook pasta according to package directions.
2. Place basil, olive oil, garlic, and pine nuts in a food processor and process until smooth. Add salt to taste.
3. Combine pesto sauce with hot cooked pasta.

For a smoother flavor, try roasting the garlic.

Spaghetti Sauce

Yield: 4 servings

1 28-oz. can tomato sauce
2 Tbs. light olive oil
2 tsp. basil
2 tsp. onion powder
1 tsp. garlic (optional)

1 tsp. oregano
salt to taste (about 1 tsp.)

1. In a 3-quart saucepan, add tomato sauce, olive oil, basil, onion powder, garlic, and oregano.
2. Bring to a low boil, reduce heat to low, cover, and simmer for 10 minutes, stirring frequently.
3. Add salt to taste.

Variation: MUSHROOM SPAGHETTI SAUCE

Sauté 2 cups sliced mushrooms with the oil. Add remaining ingredients and simmer for 10 minutes.

Variation: ITALIAN SAUSAGE SPAGHETTI SAUCE

Cut up one 14-oz. package vegan Italian sausage links. Sauté sausage with ½ diced onion in the oil until sausage is browned. Add remaining ingredients and simmer for 10 minutes.

Makes enough sauce for 12 oz. (uncooked) pasta.

Spanikopita

Yield: 6 servings

1 16-oz. package phyllo dough, thawed
1 onion, diced
3 Tbs. light olive oil
1 bunch fresh spinach, chopped
1½ tsp. salt
2 tsp. onion powder

1 tsp. garlic
¼ tsp. nutmeg
¼ tsp. black pepper
2½ Tbs. lemon juice
1 pound firm tofu
¼ cup light olive oil or more

* Preheat oven to 350°F.

1. In a 3-quart saucepan, sauté the onion in the olive oil until tender.
2. Add spinach, salt, onion powder, garlic, nutmeg, pepper, and lemon juice. Sauté until spinach is wilted.
3. Transfer contents of saucepan to a food processor. Add tofu. Process until smooth.
4. On a dry surface, stack 5 sheets of phyllo dough, lightly brushing oil on each one.
5. Cut the sheets into 4½ x 13-inch strips.
6. Place ¼ cup of filling on the top of each strip.
7. Flag fold the strips corner to corner to seal in the filling.
8. Place on a cookie sheet.
9. Repeat steps 4–8 until all of the filling is used.
10. Lightly brush the top of each pastry with olive oil.
11. Bake for 15 minutes or until golden brown.

This dish can be served as an
entrée or made smaller and
served as an appetizer.

Curry Baked Tofu

Yield: 3 servings

3 cups cooked jasmine rice* (p. 96)
3 Tbs. flour
3 Tbs. light olive oil
1 tsp. curry powder
⅛ tsp. cinnamon

¾ tsp. salt
½ cup apple juice
1 14-oz. can unsweetened coconut milk
16 oz. pressed tofu

*Substitute brown rice or couscous if you prefer.

* Preheat oven to 375°F.

1. In a 3-quart saucepan, combine flour, oil, curry, cinnamon, and salt. Cook on stove top, on medium heat, until it starts to bubble, stirring frequently.
2. Add apple juice and coconut milk.
3. Heat sauce to a low boil, stirring frequently.
4. Pour ½ of the curry sauce into a 9 x 13-inch baking dish. Place tofu on top of curry sauce. Cover the tofu with remaining sauce.
5. Bake, uncovered, for 30 minutes.
6. Serve over a bed of rice.

A smooth-flavored curry dish.

Red Curry Soba Noodle Casserole

Yield: 5 servings

1 14-oz. can unsweetened coconut milk
1 Tbs. red curry paste*
1 Tbs. sesame oil
¼ cup soy sauce**
¼ cup water
¼ cup peanut, almond, or soy butter
3 7-oz. packages fresh soba noodles***
2 cups bite-sized broccoli pieces
1 2-oz. jar diced pimientos

Optional Garnish:
¼ cup toasted coconut (p. 299)
¼ cup chopped roasted salted peanuts

*Substitute ½ tsp. dried curry powder if you prefer.
**Substitute Bragg liquid aminos if you prefer.
***Substitute 12 oz. cooked spaghetti if you prefer.

* Preheat oven to 350°F.

1. Boil soba noodles for 3 minutes. Drain off water and set noodles aside.
2. In a large bowl, whisk together the coconut milk, red curry paste, sesame oil, soy sauce, water, and nut butter. Stir in the soba noodles, broccoli, and pimientos.
3. Transfer to a 9 x 13-inch baking dish.
4. Bake, covered, for 30 minutes.
5. Garnish with coconut and peanuts.

Thai Curry Potatoes

Yield: 6 servings

3 large russet potatoes, peeled and cut into
    ¾-inch cubes
3 Tbs. light olive oil
½ onion, diced
6 mushrooms, sliced
1 small bunch spinach, chopped

⅓ cup flour
1 tsp. curry powder
⅛ tsp. cayenne pepper (optional)
2 cups vegetable broth
1 14-oz. can unsweetened coconut milk
salt to taste (about 1½ tsp.)

1. Boil potatoes until just tender, about 10 minutes. Drain off water and set potatoes aside.
2. In a large stockpot, sauté the onions and mushrooms in the oil until tender. Reduce heat to low.
3. On reduced heat, add spinach, flour, curry, and cayenne pepper. Continue cooking until spinach is wilted.
4. Turn up heat to medium. Add vegetable broth, coconut milk, and potatoes. Cook until hot and thickened, stirring frequently.
5. Simmer for 5 minutes, stirring occasionally.
6. Add salt to taste.

Serve over rice or couscous if you like.

Thai Grilled Tofu over Coconut Rice

Yield: 4 servings

4 cups cooked coconut jasmine rice (p. 92)
1 pound pressed tofu (p. 294)

Marinade:
Zest of one lime, minced
Juice of one lime
¼ cup dark sesame oil
2 Tbs. seasoned rice vinegar
2 Tbs. soy sauce
1 Tbs. sugar

Sauté mix:
3 Tbs. dark sesame oil
½ pound fresh green beans, stemmed
1 red bell pepper, small julienne cut
½ onion, small julienne cut
2 medium carrots, small julienne cut
1 cup frozen soybeans
2 Tbs. soy sauce

1. Blend all marinade ingredients until smooth. Reserve ¼ of the marinade for final drizzling of finished dish.
2. Marinate pressed tofu in remaining marinade for 4–12 hours.
3. On a flat-top grill, grill tofu until browned on each side. Cut into strips.
4. With the sesame oil, sauté the green beans, pepper, onion, carrots, and soybeans until they are tender but still a bit crisp. Add soy sauce.
5. Serve sautéed vegetables and sliced tofu over rice. Top with a small drizzle of reserved marinade.

A great-looking presentation of this dish will make it a fine choice for company.

Biryani

2 Tbs. light olive oil
1 red bell pepper, diced
1 carrot, diced
½ onion, diced
1 tsp. turmeric
¾ tsp. garlic (optional)
½ tsp. cinnamon
½ tsp. cumin
¼ tsp. ginger

⅛ tsp. cayenne (optional)
1 cup uncooked basmati rice
2 cups water
½ cup frozen peas
½ cup raisins
salt to taste (about ½ tsp.)
¾ cup whole roasted salted cashews

1. In a 3-quart saucepan, sauté the onion, carrot, and pepper in the oil until tender. Reduce heat to low.
2. On reduced heat, add the garlic, turmeric, cinnamon, cumin, ginger, and cayenne pepper. Sauté for 2 more minutes.
3. Add rice and water. On medium/high heat, bring mixture to a boil, stirring often. Reduce heat to low, cover, and simmer for 25 minutes or until rice is tender.
4. Add peas and raisins. Cover and let stand for 5 minutes.
5. Add salt to taste.
6. Garnish with cashews.

Eggplant Sauce over Rice

Yield: 4 servings

4 cups cooked basmati rice* (p. 89)
3 Tbs. light olive oil
1 sweet white onion, diced
4 cloves garlic, minced
1¼ cups canned artichoke hearts (drained)
1 eggplant, peeled and diced

1 tomato, diced
1 Tbs. garam masala
½ tsp. cinnamon
½ tsp. cumin
⅛ tsp. cayenne pepper (optional)
salt to taste (about 2 tsp.)

*Substitute brown rice if you prefer.

1. In a 3-quart saucepan, sauté the onion and garlic in the oil until tender. Reduce heat to low.
2. On reduced heat, add artichoke hearts, eggplant, tomato, garam masala, cinnamon, and cumin. Cover and simmer for 15 minutes.
3. Add salt to taste.

Eggplant is a popular choice for many Indian dishes.

Indian Lentils over Rice

Yield: 5 servings

4 cups cooked basmati rice* (p. 89)
1 cup raw green lentils, rinsed
4 cups water
3 cups vegetable broth**
3 Tbs. light olive oil
2 ribs celery, diced
½ onion, diced

1 red bell pepper, diced
1 bunch spinach, chopped
1 Tbs. curry powder
¼ cup flour
⅓ cup tomato paste
salt to taste (about 1½ tsp.)

*Substitute brown rice if you prefer.
**If using the homemade vegetable broth on p. 300, you may need to add salt to this recipe.

1. Soak the lentils in the 4 cups of water for 1 hour, or overnight in the refrigerator.
2. Drain off water and rinse lentils.
3. In a large pot, add lentils and vegetable broth. Bring to a boil, reduce heat to low, cover, and simmer for 45 minutes or until lentils are tender, stirring frequently.
4. In a 3-quart saucepan, sauté the celery, onion, and bell pepper in the oil until tender. Reduce heat to low.
5. On reduced heat, add the spinach, curry, flour, and tomato paste. Sauté for 2 more minutes.
6. Add the sautéed vegetable mixture to the cooked lentils.
7. Bring to a boil, reduce heat to low, and simmer for 5 minutes, stirring frequently.
8. Add salt to taste.
9. Serve over a bed of rice.

Tomato Garam Masala with Garbanzo Beans

Yield: 5 servings

4 cups cooked basmati rice* (p. 89)
1 bell pepper, diced
½ onion, diced
3 Tbs. light olive oil
1 tsp. garam masala
1 tsp. curry powder

1 tsp. sugar
1 28-oz. can crushed tomatoes
1 15-oz. can garbanzo beans, drained and
    rinsed
salt to taste (about 1½ tsp.)

*Substitute brown rice if you prefer.

1. In a 3-quart saucepan, sauté the pepper and onion in the oil until tender. Reduce heat to low.
2. On reduced heat, add garam masala, curry powder, and sugar. Continue to sauté for 2 minutes.
3. Add tomatoes and garbanzo beans to sautéed mix. Turn heat back up and cook sauce until hot, stirring frequently.
4. Reduce heat and simmer for 10 minutes.
5. Add salt to taste.
6. Serve over rice.

Indian dishes provide wholesome and satisfying meals.

Asian Noodles

3 7-oz. packages fresh soba noodles*
3 Tbs. sesame oil
½ onion, diced
1 red bell pepper, diced
1 bunch broccoli, cut into bite-sized pieces

¼ cup soy sauce**
¼ cup diced green onions

*Substitute 12 oz. cooked spaghetti if you prefer.
**Substitute Bragg liquid aminos if you prefer.

1. Boil soba noodles for 3 minutes. Drain off water and set noodles aside.
2. In a large pan, sauté onion, pepper, and broccoli with sesame oil until tender.
3. Stir in noodles and soy sauce and sauté until hot.
4. Garnish with green onions.

Entrée-Style Fried Rice

Yield: 4 servings

1 cup brown rice
2 cups vegetable broth
2 Tbs. sesame oil
6 mushrooms, small dice
2 ribs celery, small dice
1 carrot, small dice
½ onion, small dice

8 oz. ready-to-serve teriyaki tofu, diced*
1 8-oz. can sliced water chestnuts, drained
1 15-oz. can cut baby corn, drained
1 5-oz. can bamboo shoots, drained
¼ cup soy sauce

*To make your own teriyaki tofu, see p. 295.

1. In a 3-quart saucepan, combine the rice and vegetable broth.
2. Bring to a boil, reduce heat to low, cover, and simmer for 45 minutes or until rice is tender.
3. Meanwhile, in a 2-quart saucepan, sauté the mushrooms, celery, carrot, and onion with the sesame oil until tender. Add tofu, water chestnuts, baby corn, bamboo shoots, and soy sauce. Heat until hot.
4. Combine the cooked rice with the sautéed vegetables.

Kung Pao Tofu

Yield: 5 servings

4 cups prepared sticky rice (p. 100)
2 Tbs. sesame oil
1 small onion, diced
5 ribs celery, diced
8 oz. ready-to-serve teriyaki tofu, large dice*
¼ cup peanut, almond, or soy butter
⅓ cup soy sauce**
1 tsp. garlic

⅛ tsp. cayenne pepper (optional)
1¼ cups cold water
2 Tbs. cornstarch

Garnish:
1 cup roasted salted or unsalted peanuts
½ cup chopped green onions

*To make your own teriyaki tofu, see p. 295.
**Substitute Bragg liquid aminos if you prefer.

1. In a 3-quart saucepan, sauté the onions and celery in the sesame oil until tender.
2. Add the tofu, nut butter, soy sauce, garlic, and cayenne pepper. Stir well.
3. In a small bowl, whisk together the cornstarch and water. Add to saucepan.
4. Over medium heat, cook until hot and thickened, stirring frequently.
5. Serve over a bed of rice. Garnish with peanuts and green onions.

This traditionally spicy dish can be toned down by leaving out the cayenne pepper.

Vegetable Stir Fry

Yield: 4 servings

4 cups cooked sticky rice (p. 100)
6 cups vegetables*
2 Tbs. sesame oil
1 cup stir-fry sauce (p. 289)
8 oz. ready-to-serve teriyaki tofu, large dice**

*Some good vegetable options are broccoli, bell peppers, carrots, onions, celery, cauliflower, mushrooms, bok choy, cabbage, pineapple, shelled soybeans, snow peas, water chestnuts, baby corn, bamboo shoots, fresh ginger, and fresh garlic.
**To make your own teriyaki tofu, see p. 295.

1. Prepare sticky rice, chop vegetables, and prepare stir-fry sauce.
2. In a large pan or wok, sauté the vegetables in the oil until tender.
3. Add stir-fry sauce and tofu and heat until hot.
4. Serve over rice.

Versatile as your imagination.

Mexican Lasagna

Yield: 6 servings

6 8-inch flour tortillas
1 16-oz. can refried beans
1 12-oz. package refrigerated soy taco filling
1 4-oz. can diced green chilies
8 oz. frozen corn

1 cup salsa
2 cups shredded cheddar or Monterey jack vegan cheese (10 oz.)

* **Preheat oven to 350°F.**

1. In a large pot or skillet, add the refried beans, taco filling, green chilies, corn, and salsa. Heat mixture on medium heat until hot, stirring frequently.
2. In an 8 x 8-inch casserole pan, layer the bean mixture, shredded cheese, and tortillas in the following order: ¼ bean mixture, ¼ cheese, 2 tortillas, ¼ bean mixture, ¼ cheese, 2 tortillas, ¼ bean mixture, ¼ cheese, 2 tortillas, ¼ bean mixture, ¼ cheese.
3. Bake, uncovered, for 20 minutes.

A festive lasagna that uses tortillas instead of pasta.

Mexican Stew Topped with Chorizo Potatoes

Yield: 6 servings

Mashed potato topping:
4 medium russet potatoes, peeled and
    quartered
12 oz. soy chorizo
½ cup soy milk
2 Tbs. light olive oil
salt to taste (about 1 tsp.)

Stew:
2 carrots, diced
1 small onion, diced
3 Tbs. light olive oil
¼ cup flour
2 cups vegetable broth
2 15-oz. cans chili

*   Preheat oven to 350°F.

Mashed potato topping:
1. Boil potatoes until soft. Drain off water and mash potatoes until smooth.
2. Stir in the soy chorizo, soy milk, and olive oil.
3. Add salt to taste.

Stew:
1. In a 3-quart saucepan, sauté the carrots and onion in the oil until tender. Reduce heat.
2. On reduced heat, add the flour and sauté for 2 more minutes, stirring frequently.
3. Turn up heat to medium. Add the vegetable broth and chili. Cook stew until hot, stirring frequently.
4. Pour stew into a 9 x 13-inch baking dish. Top with mashed potato topping.
5. Bake, uncovered, for 10 minutes.

Mexican-Style Stuffed Peppers

Yield: 4 servings

1 cup uncooked brown rice
2 cups vegetable broth
4 bell peppers
2 Tbs. light olive oil
½ onion, diced
1 4-oz. can diced green chilies

½ cup salsa
½ cup frozen corn
½ cup shredded vegan cheddar cheese
1 tsp. salt

*   Preheat oven to 425°F.

1. In 2-quart saucepan, combine rice and water. Bring to a boil, cover, reduce heat to low and simmer for 45 minutes or until rice is tender.
2. Cut peppers in half from top to bottom. Remove stems and seeds.
3. Place peppers in a baking dish and cook, uncovered, for 25 minutes.
4. In a 3-quart saucepan, sauté the onion in the oil until tender.
5. Add the green chilies, salsa, corn, cheese, salt, and cooked rice.
6. Stuff peppers with rice mixture.
7. Return stuffed peppers to oven and bake, uncovered, for 10 minutes.

Variation: CHIPOTLE STUFFED PEPPERS
Add 2 Tbs. diced canned chipotle peppers to the sautéed onions.

Tamale Pie

Yield: Two 9-inch pies

Corn bread batter (p. 211)
1 bell pepper, diced
½ onion, diced
2 Tbs. light olive oil
1 4-oz. can diced green chilies
1½ cups frozen corn

1 12-oz. package refrigerated soy taco filling
2 tsp. chili powder
1 tsp. salt

* **Preheat oven to 400°F.**

1. Prepare corn bread batter and set aside.
2. In a large pan, sauté the bell pepper and onion in the oil until tender.
3. Add green chilies, corn, soy taco filling, chili powder, and salt.
4. Heat until hot, stirring frequently.
5. Pour mixture into two 9-inch round pie dishes.
6. Pour corn bread batter on top of the tamale pie filling.
7. Bake, uncovered, for 20 minutes or until toothpick inserted in the center of the corn bread comes out clean.

Mexican pie with corn bread crust topping.

Beverages

(Smoothies, Cold Beverages, and Hot Beverages)

Banana Smoothie

Yield: 3 servings

3 bananas, sliced
10 ice cubes
1½ cups soy milk
3 Tbs. sugar
1 Tbs. vanilla

Place all ingredients in a blender and blend until smooth.

Variation: NO SUGAR ADDED BANANA SMOOTHIE
For sugar, substitute powdered stevia extract to taste, about ⅛ to ¼ teaspoon.

Cream Soda Mango Smoothie

Yield: 4 servings

1 12-oz. can vanilla cream soda
1 cup soy milk
4 cups chilled or frozen mango chunks (12 oz.)

In a blender, blend all ingredients until smooth.

Mango Smoothie

Yield: 4 servings

3 cups chilled or frozen mango chunks
2½ cups soy milk
¼ cup sugar
1 tsp. vanilla
¾ tsp. coconut extract (optional)

Place all ingredients in a blender and blend until smooth.

Variation: NO SUGAR ADDED MANGO SMOOTHIE

For sugar, substitute ¼ tsp. powered stevia extract.

Mango smoothies go well with spicy Indian food.

Orange Smoothie

Yield: 4 servings

2½ cups ice cubes
2 cups soy milk
1 cup frozen orange juice concentrate
1 tsp. vanilla

Place all ingredients in a blender and blend until smooth.

Peach Tea Smoothie

¾ cup water
5 peach tea bags
1 6-oz. soy yogurt (plain, vanilla, or peach)
2 cups chilled or frozen peaches, chopped
¼ cup sugar
7 ice cubes

1. In a small saucepan, bring water to a boil. Remove from heat and add tea bags. Let tea steep for 3 minutes. Squeeze out tea bags into the tea, and then discard the tea bags.
2. In a blender, blend the tea, yogurt, peaches, sugar, and ice cubes until smooth.

Variation: NO SUGAR ADDED PEACH TEA SMOOTHIE
For sugar, substitute ¼ tsp. powdered stevia extract.

Pineapple Banana Smoothie

Yield: 4 servings

1½ cups chilled or frozen pineapple tidbits
2 ripe bananas, sliced
10 ice cubes
1½ cups soy milk
1 6-oz. soy yogurt (plain, vanilla, or peach)

¼ cup sugar
1 tsp. vanilla

Place all ingredients in a blender and blend until smooth.

Variation: NO SUGAR ADDED PINEAPPLE BANANA SMOOTHIE
For sugar, substitute ¼ tsp. powered stevia extract.

Eggless Nog

12⅓ oz. silken tofu (about 1½ cups)
2½ cups soy milk
¾ cup sugar
½ tsp. nutmeg
1 tsp. vanilla

1. In a blender, blend tofu, soy milk, sugar, nutmeg, and vanilla.
2. Serve chilled.

Variation: REDUCED-SUGAR EGGLESS NOG
Reduce sugar to ¼ cup and add ½ tsp. powdered stevia extract.

Variation: NO SUGAR ADDED EGGLESS NOG
For sugar, substitute ½ tsp. powdered stevia extract.

For a real treat, use freshly grated nutmeg.

Quick Eggless Nog

Yield: 1 serving

1 cup soy milk
1 Tbs. sugar
⅛ tsp. nutmeg

In a mug, stir all ingredients together.

Variation: NO SUGAR ADDED QUICK EGGLESS NOG
For sugar, substitute dash of powdered stevia extract.

Grandma's Ginger Beer

Yield: 10 servings

2 cups chopped fresh unpeeled ginger
2 cups sugar
2 cups water
juice of 1 lime
juice of 1 lemon
8 cups club soda

1. Place ginger, sugar, water, lime juice, and lemon juice in a blender, and blend for 15 seconds.
2. Pour into a large glass jar and put on lid.
3. Place jar in the sun for 8 hours.
4. Strain out the ginger, keeping the liquid and discarding the ginger.
5. Place beer in the refrigerator until chilled.
6. To serve, pour ¼ cup beer and ¾ cup club soda into a glass over ice.

Variation: GINGER BEER, COOKED METHOD
Place ginger mixture in a large pot instead of a glass jar. Skip steps 2 & 3. Bring to a boil, reduce heat to low, cover, and simmer for 1 hour. Continue with steps 4, 5, & 6.

Nonalcoholic.

Lemonade

Yield: 8 servings

1 cup fresh-squeezed lemon juice (about 6 lemons)
7 cups water
1 cup sugar
ice cubes

1. Combine lemon juice, water, and sugar.
2. Serve over ice.

Variation: REDUCED-SUGAR LEMONADE
Reduce sugar to ½ cup and add ½ tsp. powdered stevia extract.

Variation: SUGAR-FREE LEMONADE
For sugar, substitute 1 tsp. powdered stevia extract.

Variation: LIMEADE
For lemon juice, substitute lime juice.

Mojitos

Yield: 4 mojitos

¼ cup packed whole mint leaves
1½ cups water
½ cup lime juice
½ cup sugar
ice cubes

¼ cup club soda
mint leaves (garnish)

1. In a small saucepan, add the ¼ cup mint leaves, water, lime juice, and sugar.
2. Bring to a boil, remove from heat, cover, and let stand for 10 minutes.
3. Strain out the mint leaves, keeping the liquid and discarding the mint.
4. Chill 15 minutes.
5. To serve, fill each glass with ice, add ½ cup of liquid and 2 Tbs. club soda.
6. Garnish with mint leaves.

**A nonalcoholic Cuban beverage.
Excellent with curry dishes
like Moroccan black bean stew.**

Party Cider

½ gallon apple juice
½ liter clear pop (like 7Up)
ice cubes

1. In a large pitcher, combine apple juice and soda.
2. Serve over ice.

Watermelon Agua Fresca

Yield: 3 servings

4 cups diced seedless watermelon
1 tsp. lemon or lime juice
2 Tbs. sugar
ice cubes

1. In a blender, blend watermelon, juice, and sugar.
2. Serve with ice.

Variation: WATERMELON AGUA FRESCA WITH MINT
Add 6 mint leaves while blending.

Chai Tea Mix

Yield: 30 cups

10 2-inch cinnamon sticks
¼ cup whole cardamom pods
2 Tbs. whole cloves
¼ tsp. aniseed
1 tsp. ground ginger
1 cup brown sugar lightly packed

¼ cup loose tea (preferably Assam or Darjeeling)

1. Place cinnamon sticks in a bag and break them into smaller pieces using a hammer.
2. In a coffee or spice grinder, finely grind the broken cinnamon sticks, cardamom pods, cloves, and anise. Place into a medium-sized bowl.
3. Add ginger, brown sugar, and loose tea.
4. Store in an airtight container.

To make one cup of tea:
1. Heat up ½ cup of water and ½ cup soy milk in a saucepan.
2. Add 1 rounded Tbs. chai tea mix and let simmer for 2 minutes.
3. Strain out spices, add additional sweetener if desired, and serve.

Variation: CHOCOLATE CHAI TEA
Add 2 tsp. chocolate syrup after tea has been strained.

Send some chai tea mix home with your guests.

Hot Chocolate

Yield: 4 cups

2 oz. unsweetened baking chocolate squares, chopped
½ cup sugar
1 tsp. vanilla
1 Tbs. light olive oil
4 cups soy milk

1. In a 3-quart saucepan, add the chocolate, sugar, vanilla, and oil. On medium/low heat, melt the chocolate mixture, stirring often.
2. While the chocolate is melting, heat up the soy milk in a separate saucepan until hot.
3. Pour the hot soy milk slowly into the saucepan with the melted chocolate mixture.
4. Turn heat up to medium/high and stir with a whisk until hot chocolate is smooth and hot.

Variation: REDUCED-SUGAR HOT CHOCOLATE
Reduce sugar to ¼ cup and add ⅛ to ¼ tsp. powered stevia extract.

Spanish Hot Chocolate

Yield: 1 and 4 servings

Single-serving recipe:
1¼ tsp. cornstarch
1 Tbs. cold water
¼ tsp. vanilla
1 Tbs. cocoa powder
2 Tbs. sugar
¾ cup soy milk

Four-serving recipe:
5 tsp. cornstarch
¼ cup cold water
1 tsp. vanilla
¼ cup cocoa powder
½ cup sugar
3 cups soy milk

1. In a medium-sized saucepan, mix together the cornstarch, water, and vanilla until cornstarch is dissolved.
2. Stir in the cocoa powder and sugar until it is a smooth paste.
3. Add soy milk. On medium/high heat, heat hot chocolate to a low boil, stirring constantly.

Variation: MEXICAN HOT CHOCOLATE
Add ⅛ tsp. cinnamon with the cocoa powder and sugar for the single-serving recipe or ½ tsp. cinnamon for the four-serving recipe.

Variation: MEXICAN HOT CHOCOLATE CALIENTE
Add a small pinch of cayenne pepper with the cocoa powder, sugar, and cinnamon for the single-serving recipe or ⅛ tsp. cayenne for the four-serving recipe.

Breads

(Yeast and Quick)

Cinnamon Rolls

Yield: 12 cinnamon rolls

1 Tbs. active dry yeast (¼-oz. package)
1 tsp. sugar
¼ cup warm water (110°F)
6 oz. silken tofu
⅓ cup sugar
½ cup extra light olive oil
½ cup soy milk
1 Tbs. vanilla

1 tsp. salt
3¼ cups flour* (divided)

Filling:
¼ cup extra light olive oil or melted margarine
1 cup brown sugar
1½ Tbs. cinnamon

*You can use half white flour and half whole wheat flour if you prefer.

1. In a large bowl, whisk together the yeast, 1 tsp. sugar, and warm water. Let stand for 5 minutes.
2. In a blender, blend the tofu, ⅓ cup sugar, ½ cup oil, soy milk, vanilla, and salt.
3. Add the contents of the blender to the contents of the large bowl and mix just until combined.
4. Whisk in 1 cup flour.
5. With a spoon, add 2¼ cups flour and stir until combined.
6. On a floured surface, knead dough for 7 minutes.
7. Place kneaded dough in a large oiled bowl, cover with a slightly damp towel or clear wrap, and let stand in a warm place for 2 hours or until doubled in size.
8. Punch down dough and knead for 1 minute.
9. On a floured surface, roll out dough to 12 x 16 inches.
10. In a small bowl, combine filling ingredients (¼ cup oil or margarine, brown sugar, and cinnamon).
11. Distribute filling mixture evenly on top of dough.
12. Roll up dough starting on the 16-inch edge.
13. Cut dough into 12 even parts. Place rolls into a lightly oiled 9 x 13-inch baking dish. Cover with a slightly damp towel or clear wrap, and let stand in a warm place for 2 hours or until doubled in size.
14. Preheat oven to 375°F.
15. Remove towel.
16. Bake for 20 minutes or until centers are no longer doughy.

Variation: WALNUT AND RAISIN CINNAMON ROLLS
Add ½ cup chopped walnuts and ½ cup raisins to the filling.

Variation: MAPLE CHUNK CINNAMON ROLLS
Reduce brown sugar to ½ cup and add 1 cup maple chunks to the filling.

Homemade Bread

Yield: 2 loaves

2 Tbs. active dry yeast (2 ¼-oz. packages)
2 tsp. sugar
¼ cup warm water (110°F)
1¾ cup warm soy milk (110°F)
2 cups flour

¼ cup extra light olive oil
2 Tbs. sugar
1 Tbs. salt
2½ cups flour (divided)

1. In a large bowl, whisk together the yeast, 2 tsp. sugar, and warm water. Let stand for 5 minutes.
2. Add soy milk, 2 cups flour, oil, 2 Tbs. sugar, and salt and whisk for 2 minutes.
3. With a spoon, add 2½ cups flour to the large bowl and stir until combined.
4. On a floured surface, knead dough for 10 minutes.
5. Place kneaded dough in a large oiled bowl, cover with a slightly damp towel, and let stand in a warm place for 2 hours or until doubled in size.
6. Punch down the dough and knead for 1 minute. Divide into 2 loaves and place in 2 oiled loaf pans.
7. Cover with a slightly damp towel and let stand in a warm place for 2 hours or until doubled in size.
8. Preheat oven to 375°F.
9. Remove towel.
10. Bake for 30 minutes or until toothpick inserted in the center comes out clean.
11. Remove from oven and cool for 5 minutes before turning onto a cooling rack. Brush top of bread with olive oil if you prefer a softer crust.

Variation: WHOLE WHEAT BREAD
Instead of 2½ cups white flour, use 2½ cups whole wheat flour.

Variation: SESAME AND FLAX SEED BREAD
For sugar, substitute 2 Tbs. molasses. Add ½ cup sesame seeds and ¼ cup ground flax seed to the dough while adding the 2½ cups flour.

Variation: HERB BREAD
With the 2½ cups flour, add 2 Tbs. basil, 1 Tbs. oregano, 2 Tbs. parsley flakes, and 1 Tbs. thyme.

Variation: POTATO "CHEESE" BREAD
With the 2½ cups flour, add 2 cups shredded potatoes, 2 cups shredded vegan cheddar cheese, and ⅛ tsp. cayenne pepper.

Pita Bread

Yield: 12

1 Tbs. active dry yeast (¼-ounce package)
1½ cups warm water (110°F)
1 tsp. sugar
1 tsp. salt
3¾ cups flour* (divided)

*You can use half white flour and half whole wheat flour if you prefer.

1. In a large bowl, whisk together the yeast, water, and sugar. Let stand for 5 minutes.
2. Whisk in the salt and 1½ cups flour.
3. With a spoon, stir in 2¼ cups flour.
4. On a lightly floured surface, knead dough for 7 minutes.
5. Place dough in an oiled bowl, cover with clear wrap, and let rise until doubled in size.
6. Punch down dough and knead for 1 minute.
7. Place a cooking stone or cookie sheet on lowest rack in oven. Remove all other racks.
8. Preheat oven to 550°F. Expect a little smoke.
9. Roll dough into a 12-inch-long rope and cut into 12 pieces.
10. On a lightly floured surface, roll each piece into 8-inch patties, about ⅛ inch thick.
11. Briefly open oven door, pull out oven rack, set one pita on stone or cookie sheet, push rack back into place, and close oven door. Pitas will bake in as little as 1½ minutes. When pitas are done baking, pull out oven rack, remove pita and place on a clean towel. Repeat until all pitas are done.

Pizza Crust

Yield: One 14-inch thick-crust pizza
or two 14-inch thin-crust pizzas

1 Tbs. active dry yeast (¼-oz. package)
1 cup warm water (110°F)
1 tsp. sugar
1 cup flour*
1 tsp. salt

¼ cup extra light olive oil
1½ cups flour

*Substitute whole wheat flour if you prefer.

1. In a large bowl, whisk together the yeast, water, and sugar. Let stand for 5 minutes.
2. Whisk in 1 cup flour, salt, and oil.
3. With a spoon, stir in 1½ cups flour.
4. On a floured surface, knead dough for 5 minutes.
5. Let dough rest for 5 minutes.
5. Roll out dough on an oiled cookie sheet or pizza stone.
6. Top with sauce and favorite toppings.
7. Let rise for 30 minutes.
8. Preheat oven to 450°F.
9. Bake for 15 minutes or until crust center is no longer doughy.

Don't forget the pizza sauce (p. 287).

Banana Bread

Yield: 1 loaf

2 cups flour*
¾ cup sugar
1 tsp. baking powder
1 tsp. egg replacer powder
½ tsp. baking soda
¾ tsp. salt

2 very ripe bananas, mashed
¼ cup soy milk
¼ cup silken tofu
¼ cup extra light olive oil
2 tsp. vanilla

*You can use half white flour and half whole wheat flour if you prefer.

*   Preheat oven to 350°F.

1. In a large bowl, whisk together the flour, sugar, baking powder, egg replacer, baking soda, and salt.
2. In a blender, blend the bananas, soy milk, tofu, oil, and vanilla until smooth.
3. Add the contents of the blender to the contents of the large bowl and mix with a spoon just until combined.
4. Spoon batter into an oiled loaf pan.
5. Bake for 55 minutes or until toothpick inserted in center comes out clean.

Variation: BANANA NUT BREAD
Add ½ cup chopped walnuts after whisking together the dry ingredients.

The best banana bread
you will ever have!

Variation: REDUCED-SUGAR BANANA BREAD
Reduce sugar to ¼ cup and add ½ tsp. powdered stevia extract.

Corn Bread

1¼ cups cornmeal
¾ cup flour*
1 Tbs. sugar
2 tsp. baking powder

2 tsp. egg replacer powder
1 tsp. salt
1¼ cups soy milk
⅓ cup extra light olive oil

* You can use half white flour and half whole wheat flour if you prefer.

* **Preheat oven to 400°F.**

1. In a large bowl, combine cornmeal, flour, sugar, baking powder, egg replacer, and salt.
2. Whisk in the soy milk and oil, and stir just until combined.
3. Pour batter into an oiled 8 x 8-inch baking dish.
4. Bake for 20 minutes or until toothpick inserted in the center comes out clean.

Variation: JALAPENO & "CHEESE" CORN BREAD
Add 4 oz shredded vegan cheddar cheese and 2 Tbs. chopped canned jalapeños.

Variation: SILKEN CORN BREAD
Reduce soy milk to 1 cup. Add ¼ cup silken tofu. In a blender, blend the soy milk, tofu, and oil. In a large bowl, add blended contents with the dry ingredients.

Flour Tortillas

Yield: Eight 8-inch tortillas

4 cups flour*
1 tsp. salt
6 oz. silken tofu
1 cup water
2 Tbs. extra light olive oil

* You can use half white flour and half whole wheat flour if you prefer.

* Preheat griddle to 425°F, or choose the medium/high setting on your stove.

1. In a large bowl, mix flour and salt.
2. In blender, blend the tofu, water, and oil.
3. Add the contents of the blender to the contents of the large bowl. Knead on a lightly floured surface until smooth, about 1 minute.
4. Divide dough into 8 pieces. Roll out dough into 8-inch rounds.
5. Place tortillas on a lightly oiled griddle or frying pan.
6. Grill on each side until lightly browned.

Zucchini Bread

Yield: 1 loaf

2 cups flour*
1 cup sugar
1½ tsp. cinnamon
¼ tsp. nutmeg
1 tsp. baking powder
1 tsp. egg replacer powder
½ tsp. baking soda

¾ tsp. salt
1 cup shredded zucchini (packed)
¼ cup silken tofu
¼ cup extra light olive oil
¼ cup soy milk
1 Tbs. vanilla extract

* You can use half white flour and half whole wheat flour if you prefer.

---

* **Preheat oven to 375°F.**

1. In a large bowl, whisk together the flour, sugar, cinnamon, nutmeg, baking powder, egg replacer, baking soda, and salt.
2. In a blender, blend the zucchini, tofu, oil, soy milk, and vanilla.
3. With a spoon, add the blended ingredients to the large bowl. Mix together until well combined. Spoon batter into an oiled loaf pan.
4. Bake for 55 minutes or until toothpick inserted in the center comes out clean.

Variation: REDUCED-SUGAR ZUCCHINI BREAD
Reduce sugar to ½ cup and add ½ tsp. powdered stevia extract.

Moist and light.

Variation: CHOCOLATE ZUCCHINI BREAD
Add ¼ cup unsweetened cocoa powder and ¾ cup chocolate chips to the dry mix.

Desserts

(Cookies, Pies, Cakes, Frostings, Puddings, and Miscellaneous desserts)

Cherry Bon Bons

Cookie dough:
12 whole maraschino cherries (reserve liquid)
½ cup margarine
¾ cup powdered sugar
1 Tbs. vanilla
⅛ tsp. salt

1½ cups flour
1 or 2 Tbs. soy milk (if needed)

Icing:
¾ cup powdered sugar
1 to 2 Tbs. maraschino cherry liquid

* Preheat oven to 350°F.

1. Cut maraschino cherries in half and place upside down on a paper towel to drain.
2. By hand, or using a food processor or mixer, combine the margarine, ¾ cup powdered sugar, vanilla, and salt until smooth. Place in a bowl and stir in flour.
3. If dough is hard to work with, add 1 or 2 Tbs. soy milk.
4. Hand-roll dough into ¾-inch balls, then press your thumb into the center to make an indention for a cherry half. Place a cherry half in center and work dough back into a ball.
5. Place on an ungreased cookie sheet.
6. Bake for 15 minutes or until lightly browned on bottom.
7. Place on a cooling rack until completely cool.
8. Make icing by combining ¾ cup powdered sugar with maraschino cherry juice. Icing should be just thick enough to cling to dipped cookies.
9. Dip tops of cookies in glaze and let set.

The best holiday cookie ever.

Chocolate Cookies

1¾ cups flour
½ cup cocoa powder
1 tsp. egg replacer powder
¾ tsp. salt
½ tsp. baking soda
1 cup sugar

⅗ cup margarine
½ cup soy milk
1 Tbs. vanilla

* **Preheat oven to 400°F.**

1. In a large bowl, whisk together the flour, cocoa powder, egg replacer, salt, and baking soda.
2. In a separate bowl or food processor, cream together the sugar, margarine, soy milk, and vanilla.
3. Stir together the sugar mixture and flour mixture.
4. Drop by rounded teaspoonfuls onto an ungreased cookie sheet. Do not flatten.
5. Bake for 11 minutes or until done. Transfer to a cooling rack when slightly cooled.

Variation: CHOCOLATE CHOCOLATE CHIP COOKIES
After combining the sugar and flour mixture, stir in 6 oz. chocolate chips.

Variation: CHOCOLATE WALNUT COOKIES
After combining the sugar and flour mixture, stir in ½ cup chopped walnuts.

Chocolate Chip Cookies

Yield: 20 cookies

1½ cups flour
1½ tsp. egg replacer powder
½ tsp. baking soda
½ tsp. salt
½ cup sugar

½ cup brown sugar*
½ cup margarine
2 Tbs. water
1 tsp. vanilla
6 oz. semisweet chocolate chips

*You can make your own brown sugar by combining ½ cup sugar with 1½ tsp. molasses.

---

*   Preheat oven to 350°F.

1. In a large bowl, whisk together the flour, egg replacer, baking soda, and salt. Set aside.
2. Cream together the sugar, brown sugar, margarine, water, and vanilla.
3. Stir together the sugar mixture and the flour mixture. You may need to use an electric mixer or food processor.
4. Add chocolate chips.
5. Drop by rounded teaspoonfuls onto an ungreased cookie sheet. Do not flatten.
6. Bake for 15 minutes or until lightly browned.

Variation: CHOCOLATE CHIP WALNUT COOKIES
Add ¾ cup chopped walnuts along with the chocolate chips.

Coconut Cookies

Yield: 24 cookies

¾ cup sugar
½ cup margarine
¼ cup water
½ tsp. baking soda
⅛ tsp. salt

3 cups unsweetened coconut flakes
1 cup flour

*   **Preheat oven to 350°F.**

1. Cream together sugar, margarine, water, baking soda, and salt.
2. Stir in the coconut flakes and flour.
3. Drop by rounded teaspoonfuls onto lightly oiled cookie sheet. Do not flatten.
4. Bake for 15 minutes or until done.

**Simple recipe,
decadent results.**

Date Sprocket Cookies

Yield: 30 cookies

Cookie dough:
2⅓ cups flour
1 Tbs. egg replacer powder
½ tsp. baking powder
¼ tsp. baking soda
¼ tsp. salt
¼ tsp. cinnamon
1 cup packed brown sugar*
½ cup margarine
¼ cup water

1 Tbs. soy milk
½ tsp. vanilla

Filling:
8 oz. pitted dates, chopped
⅓ cup sugar
⅓ cup water
½ cup finely chopped walnuts
½ tsp. vanilla

*You can make your own brown sugar by combining 1 cup of sugar with 1 Tbs. molasses.

1. In a large bowl, whisk together the flour, egg replacer, baking powder, baking soda, salt, and cinnamon.
2. Cream together the sugar, margarine, water, soy milk, and vanilla.
3. Stir together the sugar mixture and flour mixture.
4. Chill dough in refrigerator for 30 minutes.
5. While dough is chilling, prepare filling. Place dates, sugar, and water in a 2-quart saucepan. Slowly bring to a boil, then simmer for 5 minutes. Remove from heat and add nuts and vanilla.
6. After cookie dough is chilled, roll out dough between two pieces of waxed paper to 10 x 18 inches. Remove and discard top piece of waxed paper.
7. Spread filling evenly on top of rolled-out dough.
8. Roll up dough into an 18-inch roll. Chill for 30 more minutes.
9. Preheat oven to 350°F.
10. Slice into ½-inch wheels and place on an oiled cookie sheet.
11. Bake for 14 minutes or until done.

These cookies are prepared like cinnamon rolls. First roll out dough, then cover with filling, roll up dough and cut into individual cookies before baking.

Double Chocolate Fudge Cookies

Yield: 36 cookies

6 oz. silken tofu
½ cup margarine
½ cup soy milk
2 tsp. vanilla
2 cups flour
2 cups sugar

½ cup cocoa powder
½ tsp. baking soda
½ tsp. baking powder
¾ tsp. salt
6 oz. semisweet chocolate chips
½ cup chopped walnuts

*   Preheat oven to 350°F.

1. In a blender, blend the tofu, margarine, soy milk, and vanilla until smooth.
2. In a large bowl, whisk together the flour, sugar, cocoa powder, baking soda, baking powder, and salt.
3. Pour the blended mixture into the flour mixture. Stir until combined.
4. Add chocolate chips and nuts.
5. Drop by rounded teaspoonfuls onto ungreased cookie sheets.
6. Bake for 15 minutes or until done.

Gingerbread Cookies

Yield: 20 5-inch gingerbread people

½ cup brown sugar*
¾ tsp. baking soda
¾ tsp. ginger
½ tsp. cinnamon
½ tsp. salt

¼ tsp. allspice
¼ tsp. cloves
½ cup molasses
⅓ cup water
2 Tbs. extra light olive oil

*You can make your own brown sugar by combining ½ cup sugar with 1½ tsp. molasses.

* Preheat oven to 350°F.

1. In a large bowl, whisk together flour, sugar, baking soda, ginger, cinnamon, salt, all-spice, and cloves.
2. With a spoon, stir in the molasses, water, and oil.
3. Knead dough until all ingredients are combined.
4. Roll out dough on a lightly floured surface to ⅛-inch thickness.
5. Cut out cookies and place on an oiled cookie sheet.
6. Bake for 11 minutes or until done. Finished cookies will be soft.

Variation: GINGERBREAD HOUSE (Yield: three 10 x 14-inch walls)

Triple gingerbread cookie recipe. Divide dough into 3 parts. Roll each part out onto an 11 x 14-inch parchment-lined cookie sheet. Bake at 350°F for 15 minutes. After gingerbread dough is cool, cut out your walls and roof pieces as needed. Let gingerbread sit out overnight, uncovered, to stiffen. Use melted sugar to join walls and roof.

MELTED SUGAR

(Melted sugar is very hot and can cause a serious burn.)

In a heavy-bottomed pan, like a cast-iron skillet, add desired amount of sugar. Over medium heat, heat sugar until liquefied, stirring frequently. Turn heat to low or remove from heat. Dip edges of gingerbread in melted sugar and attach to desired location. Hold until secured. Sugar can be reheated a couple of times.

Lemon Nutty Biscotti

Yield: 30 cookies

6 oz. silken tofu
1 cup sugar
⅓ cup extra light olive oil
zest of 2 lemons
3 Tbs. lemon juice
1 tsp. vanilla

2 cups flour*
1 cup semolina flour
1 tsp. baking soda
1 tsp. baking powder
½ cup chopped almonds
½ tsp. salt

*You can use half white flour and half whole wheat flour if you prefer.

* Preheat oven to 375°F.

1. In a food processor or blender, combine tofu, sugar, oil, zest, lemon juice, and vanilla.
2. In a large bowl, whisk together the flours, baking soda, baking powder, almonds, and salt.
3. Stir tofu mixture into flour mixture.
4. On an oiled cookie sheet, form dough into two 12-inch-long logs.
5. Bake for 25 minutes.
6. Remove from oven and cool on counter for 15 minutes.
7. Reduce oven temperature to 300°F.
8. Slice logs into ¾-inch slices and lay slices flat on ungreased cookie sheets.
9. Bake for 40 minutes, turning cookies once after 20 minutes. Additional cooking time may be added for an even crunchier cookie.

Lime Cookies

Yield: 48 cookies

¾ cup margarine
⅓ cup powdered sugar
zest of two limes
2 Tbs. lime juice
1 Tbs. vanilla
2 Tbs. cornstarch

¼ tsp. salt
2 cups flour
¾ cup powdered sugar (for coating)

1. Cream together margarine, ⅓ cup powdered sugar, lime zest, lime juice, vanilla, cornstarch, and salt.
2. Stir in flour.
3. Roll dough into two logs, 1¼ inches in diameter. Place logs between two pieces of parchment or waxed paper and place in freezer for 1 hour.
4. Preheat oven to 350°F.
5. Remove dough from freezer and cut into ¼-inch rounds. Place on parchment-lined or oiled cookie sheet.
6. Bake for 15 minutes or until done. Cool slightly on a cooling rack.
7. Gently toss all slightly cooled cookies in powdered sugar one at a time, then toss in powdered sugar a second time.

Molasses Crinkle Tops

Yield: 40 cookies

1 cup sugar
¾ cup margarine
¼ cup molasses
1½ tsp. egg replacer powder
2 Tbs. water
2 cups flour

2 tsp. baking soda
½ tsp. ground cloves
½ tsp. salt
½ tsp. ground ginger
1 cup raisins
½ cup sugar (for rolling cookies in)

* Preheat oven to 350°F.

1. Cream together sugar, margarine, molasses, egg replacer, and water.
2. In a large bowl, whisk together the flour, baking soda, cloves, salt, and ginger.
3. Stir in sugar mixture.
4. Add raisins.
5. Form into walnut-sized balls, roll in sugar, and place on an ungreased cookie sheet, leaving room for cookies to spread. No need to flatten the cookies before baking.
6. Bake for 14 minutes or until done. These cookies are better a little undercooked than overcooked, so watch them carefully.

The raisins really make this recipe.

Chewy Oatmeal Cookies

Yield: 24 cookies

2½ cups quick oatmeal (uncooked)
1 cup flour
¾ tsp. salt
½ tsp. baking soda
¾ cup margarine
1 cup brown sugar*

½ cup sugar
6 Tbs. water
1½ tsp. egg replacer powder
1 tsp. vanilla

*You can make your own brown sugar by combining 1 cup of sugar with 1 Tbs. molasses.

*   Preheat oven to 350°F.

1. In a large bowl, whisk together the oatmeal, flour, salt, and baking soda.
2. In a separate bowl, cream together margarine, brown sugar, sugar, water, egg replacer, and vanilla.
3. Combine creamed ingredients with oatmeal mixture.
4. Drop by rounded teaspoonfuls onto an ungreased cookie sheet. Flatten slightly.
5. Bake for 15 minutes or until lightly browned.

Variation: OATMEAL CHOCOLATE CHIP COOKIES
Add ¾ cup chocolate chips with the oatmeal.

Variation: OATMEAL RAISIN COOKIES
Add ¾ cup raisins and 1 tsp. cinnamon with the oatmeal.

Orange Zest & Crystallized Ginger Cookies

Yield: 44 cookies

1¼ cups blanched almonds
1 cup powdered sugar
¾ cup margarine
3 Tbs. orange zest
2 Tbs. water
1½ tsp. egg replacer powder

1 Tbs. orange juice
1½ cups flour
½ cup chopped crystallized ginger

1. Place almonds and sugar in a food processor. Process until mixture resembles coarse crumbs.
2. Add margarine, orange zest, water, egg replacer, and orange juice. Process until smooth.
3. In a large bowl, combine the flour and ginger.
4. Add the almond mixture to the flour mixture. Stir until well mixed.
5. Between two 8 x 12-inch pieces of waxed or parchment paper, roll dough into two logs, 1¼ inches in diameter. Chill 1 hour.
6. Preheat oven to 350°F.
7. Remove paper and slice logs into ½-inch rounds. Place on oiled cookie sheet.
8. Bake for 15 minutes or until done.

Peanut Butter Cookies

Yield: 24 cookies

1¾ cups flour
½ tsp. baking soda
½ tsp. salt
¾ cup pure maple syrup
¼ cup sugar
¼ cup margarine

¾ cup peanut butter
1 Tbs. vanilla

---

*   Preheat oven to 350°F.

1.   In a large bowl, whisk together flour, baking soda, and salt.
2.   In a separate bowl, cream together the maple syrup, sugar, margarine, peanut butter, and vanilla.
3.   Stir together sugar mixture and flour mixture.
4.   Drop by rounded teaspoonfuls onto a lightly oiled cookie sheet. Flatten with the tines of a fork.
5.   Bake for 14 minutes or until done.

Variation: PEANUT BUTTER CHOCOLATE CHIP COOKIES

After combining sugar mixture and flour mixture, stir in ¾ cup chocolate chips.

Variation: ALMOND BUTTER COOKIES

Substitute almond butter for peanut butter.

Variation: SOY BUTTER COOKIES

Substitute soy butter for peanut butter.

Creamy or chunky peanut butter, it's your choice.

Pumpkin Cookies

Yield: 48 cookies

2 cups flour
1 cup sugar
1 tsp. baking powder
1 tsp. baking soda
1 tsp. cinnamon
¼ tsp. salt

1 cup canned pumpkin
½ cup extra light olive oil
½ cup raisins

*   Preheat oven to 375°F.

1. In a large bowl, whisk together the flour, sugar, baking powder, baking soda, cinnamon, and salt.
2. Add pumpkin and oil.
3. Add raisins.
4. Drop by rounded teaspoonfuls onto a lightly oiled cookie sheet.
5. Bake for 10 minutes or until done.

Variation: SILKEN PUMPKIN COOKIES
For olive oil, substitute ½ cup silken tofu. Use a food processor or blender to mix tofu with pumpkin.

Soft, moist cookies.

Snicker Doodles

Yield: 36 cookies

3 cups flour*
1½ cups sugar
1 Tbs. egg replacer powder
2 tsp. cream of tartar
1 tsp. baking soda
½ tsp. salt

¾ cup soy milk
½ cup margarine, softened**
1 tsp. vanilla
¼ cup sugar
2 tsp. cinnamon

*You can use half white flour and half whole wheat flour if you prefer.
**Substitute light olive oil if you prefer.

* Preheat oven to 400°F.

1. In a large bowl, whisk together flour, 1½ cups sugar, egg replacer, cream of tartar, baking soda, and salt.
2. Stir in soy milk, margarine, and vanilla.
3. In a separate bowl, combine ¼ cup sugar and cinnamon.
4. Roll dough into 1-inch balls. Roll balls in cinnamon and sugar and place on an oiled cookie sheet.
5. Bake for 10 minutes or until lightly browned on bottom.

Sugar Cookies

Yield: 30 cookies

1½ cups powdered sugar
1 cup margarine
2 Tbs. water
1 tsp. vanilla
½ tsp. almond extract
2½ cups flour

1½ tsp. egg replacer powder
1 tsp. baking soda
1 tsp. cream of tartar

1. Cream together powdered sugar, margarine, water, vanilla, and almond extract.
2. In a separate bowl, mix the flour, egg replacer, baking soda, and cream of tartar.
3. Mix creamed sugar mixture with flour mixture.
4. Chill in airtight container for at least 2 hours.
5. Preheat oven to 375°F.
6. Roll out dough on a lightly floured surface to ⅛-inch thickness.
7. Cut out cookies and place on lightly oiled or parchment-lined cookie sheet.
8. Bake for 7 minutes or until done.

Walnut Cookies

1 cup margarine
1½ cups powdered sugar (divided)
1 tsp. vanilla
2¼ cups flour
¼ tsp. salt
¾ cup finely chopped walnuts

*   Preheat oven to 400°F.

1. By hand, food processor, or mixer, combine margarine, ½ cup powdered sugar, vanilla, flour, and salt.
2. Transfer to a large bowl and stir in the walnuts.
3. Roll into 1-inch balls.
4. Place on ungreased cookie sheet.
5. Bake until set but not brown, approximately 10–12 minutes.
6. Cool for 5 minutes.
7. Roll cookies in 1 cup powdered sugar once, then a second time.

Single Pie Crust

Yield: One 9-inch pie crust

1¾ cups flour
1 tsp. salt
½ cup extra light olive oil
3 Tbs. cold water

1. In a large bowl, thoroughly mix the flour and salt.
2. Stir in the oil and water with a dinner fork just until combined. Do not overwork pastry.
3. Roll dough out between two pieces of waxed paper or on a lightly floured surface to desired size.

When a recipe calls for a precooked pie crust:

1. Place pie crust in desired pie dish.
2. Prick bottom and sides of crust with a fork.
3. Bake at 425°F for 10 minutes.

This pie crust recipe can be used for a double pie crust if you divide the prepared dough in two and roll out thinly.

Double Pie Crust

Yield: Two 9-inch pie crusts

2⅗ cups flour
1½ tsp. salt
¾ cup extra light olive oil
¼ cup cold water

1. In a large bowl, thoroughly mix the flour and salt.
2. Stir in the oil and water with a dinner fork just until combined. Do not overwork pastry.
3. Divide dough into 2 dough balls. Roll each dough ball between two pieces of waxed paper or on a lightly floured surface to desired size.

> **This recipe will give you two thick pie crusts so you will have a top and bottom crust for your pie. If you prefer thin crusts you can use the single pie crust recipe.**

Citrus Pie Crust

Yield: One 9-inch pie crust

2 cups flour
2 Tbs. sugar
3 tsp. fresh lemon, orange, or lime zest
1 tsp. salt
½ cup extra light olive oil
¼ cup lemon, orange, or lime juice

1. In a large bowl, thoroughly mix the flour, sugar, zest, and salt.
2. Add the oil and juice and stir with a dinner fork just until combined. Do not overwork pastry.
3. Roll dough out between two pieces of waxed paper or on a lightly floured surface to desired size.

Graham Cracker Pie Crust

Yield: One 9-inch pie crust

10 whole graham crackers
4 Tbs. margarine, softened
3 Tbs. sugar

If you have a food processor:
1. Grind crackers in food processor to fine crumbs.
2. Add margarine and sugar and blend until combined.
3. Press crumbs into the bottom of pie dish and up the sides.
4. Chill in refrigerator before filling.

If you don't have a food processor:
1. Place crackers in a plastic bag and crush with a rolling pin.
2. Pour crumbs into a large bowl.
3. Stir in margarine and sugar until well combined.
4. Press crumbs into the bottom of pie dish and up the sides.
5. Chill in refrigerator before filling.

Apple Pie

Yield: One 9-inch pie

---

6 cups peeled and cored apple slices
¾ cup sugar
¼ cup flour
1 tsp. cinnamon
½ tsp. nutmeg

9-inch double pie crust (p. 234)

---

*   Preheat oven to 425°F.

1. In a large bowl, combine apples, sugar, flour, cinnamon, and nutmeg.
2. Prepare pie crust. Line bottom of pie dish with bottom crust.
3. Pour apples into pie dish.
4. Cover with top crust and seal edges. Cut a few slits in top crust.
5. Bake for 45 minutes or until juice begins to bubble.

Variation: REDUCED-SUGAR APPLE PIE
Reduce sugar to ¼ cup and add ½ tsp. powdered stevia extract.

Cherry Pie

4 cups fresh or frozen (thawed) pitted pie
    cherries and their juice
3 Tbs. minute tapioca granules
1 cup sugar
⅛ tsp. almond extract

1 Tbs. margarine
9-inch double pie crust (p. 234)

*   Preheat oven to 425°F.

1. In a large bowl, combine cherries, tapioca, sugar, and almond extract. Let soak while preparing pie crust, stirring occasionally.
2. Prepare pie crust and line bottom of pie dish with bottom crust.
3. Pour cherries into pie dish.
4. Dot top of cherries with margarine.
5. Cover with top crust and seal edges. Cut a few slits in top crust.
6. Bake for 45 minutes or until juice begins to bubble.

Variation: REDUCED-SUGAR CHERRY PIE
Reduce sugar to ¾ cup and add ½ tsp. powdered stevia extract.

Chocolate Cream Pie

Yield: One 9-inch pie

9-inch precooked single pie crust (p. 233)
or 9-inch graham cracker crust (p. 236)
2 12⅓-oz. packages silken tofu (about 3
    cups)
1½ cups powdered sugar

2 Tbs. vanilla extract
3 cups chocolate chips

1. Prepare pie crust of choice and set aside.
2. In a food processor, combine tofu, sugar, and vanilla until smooth. Leave mixture in food processor.
3. In a double boiler, melt chocolate chips until just smooth and melted.
4. With food processor on, slowly drizzle in the melted chocolate. Process until well mixed, scraping down sides as needed.
5. Pour chocolate mixture into prepared crust.
6. Refrigerate until set.

Variation: CHOCOLATE COCONUT CREAM PIE

By hand, stir in 1¼ cups shredded unsweetened coconut after the melted chocolate has been added.

For a cool summer treat, try serving this pie frozen.

Cobbler-Crusted Apple Pie

Yield: One 9-inch pie

4 large apples, peeled, cored, and ¼-inch
    sliced
⅓ cup sugar
½ tsp. cinnamon
⅓ cup margarine, melted and cooled to
    room temperature

1 cup flour
½ cup sugar
½ cup brown sugar
1 tsp. baking powder
¾ cup soy milk

*   Preheat oven to 375°F.

1. In a medium-sized bowl, combine apples, ⅓ cup sugar, and cinnamon. Set aside.
2. Pour melted margarine into a 9-inch pie dish and tilt dish to coat sides with margarine.
3. In a medium-sized bowl, whisk together the flour, ½ cup sugar, brown sugar, and baking powder.
4. Stir in soy milk.
5. Slowly pour batter evenly over butter in pie dish.
6. Neatly arrange apple mixture on top of batter.
7. Bake for 50 minutes or until dough is cooked in the center.

**A sweet, biscuit-style,
crusted apple pie.**

Coconut Cream Pie

Yield: One 9-inch pie

Coconut pudding* (p. 261)
Graham cracker crust (p. 236)
2 Tbs. toasted coconut (optional) (p. 299)

*If using the recipe on p. 261, you may have some filling left over.

1. Place pudding in the refrigerator for 15 minutes to cool.
2. Pour into prepared pie crust.
3. Chill until set.
4. Garnish with toasted coconut.

Key Lime Pie

Yield: One 9-inch pie

12⅓ oz. silken tofu (about 1½ cups)
8 oz. vegan cream cheese
½ cup lime juice
2 packages Morinu Tofu Mate vanilla pud-
　　ding mix
4 tsp. sugar

1 single precooked 9-inch pie crust (p. 233)
　　or graham cracker crust (p. 236)

1. In a food processor, combine tofu, cream cheese, lime juice, pudding mix, and sugar.
2. Pour into prepared pie crust.
3. Chill until set, about 4 hours.

Pecan Pie

Yield: One 9-inch pie

2 cups toasted pecan halves, chopped by
    hand or in food processor
¾ cup + 2 Tbs. sugar
½ cup water
2 tsp. cornstarch or arrowroot
2 tsp. vanilla

pinch of salt
9-inch single pie crust (p. 233)

*   Preheat oven to 425°F.

1.   In a medium-sized bowl, combine all ingredients.
2.   Pour into pastry-lined pie dish.
3.   Bake 20 to 25 minutes or until crust is lightly browned and filling is bubbling.

Pumpkin Pie

Yield: One 9-inch pie

12⅓ oz. silken tofu (about 1½ cups)
¾ cup + 2 Tbs. sugar
2 cups canned pumpkin* (15-oz. can)
1½ tsp. cinnamon
¾ tsp. ginger

½ tsp. salt
¼ tsp. nutmeg
⅛ tsp. cloves

9-inch single pie crust (p. 233)

*Substitute fresh pumpkin, yams, or sweet potato if you prefer.

---

* Preheat oven to 350°F.

1. In a food processor, blend the tofu, sugar, pumpkin, cinnamon, ginger, salt, nutmeg, and cloves. Process until smooth.
2. Prepare pie crust. Line bottom of pie dish with crust.
3. Pour pumpkin mixture into dish.
4. Bake for 1 hour.
5. Chill, uncovered, in refrigerator before serving.

Variation: REDUCED-SUGAR PUMPKIN PIE
Reduce sugar to 6 Tbs. and add ½ tsp. powdered
stevia extract.

**Enjoy pumpkin pie year round
with this easy recipe.**

Rhubarb Pie

Yield: One 9-inch pie

6 cups cut-up rhubarb (½-inch pieces)
1¼ cups sugar
¼ cup flour
2 tsp. cornstarch

9-inch double pie crust (p. 234)

*   Preheat oven to 425°F.

1. In a large bowl, combine rhubarb, sugar, flour, and cornstarch. Toss until rhubarb is coated.
2. Prepare pie crust and line bottom of pie dish with bottom crust.
3. Toss rhubarb mix once more before pouring into pie dish.
4. Cover with top crust and seal edges. Cut a few slits in top crust.
5. Bake for 50 minutes or until juice begins to bubble.

Variation: REDUCED-SUGAR RHUBARB PIE
Reduce sugar to ¾ cup and add ½ tsp. powdered stevia extract.

Black Forest Cake

Yield: Two 8-inch rounds or one 9 x 13-inch cake

2 cups cake flour

1½ cups sugar

⅗ cup unsweetened baking cocoa powder

1 Tbs. egg replacer powder

1 tsp. baking soda

½ tsp. salt

⅗ cup chopped nuts

1½ cups pitted chopped dark sweet cherries (fresh, canned, or frozen and thawed)

1 cup soy milk

6 Tbs. extra light olive oil

2 tsp. vanilla

chocolate frosting (p. 253) (optional)

* Preheat oven to 350°F.

1. Oil and flour cake pan(s).
2. In a large bowl, whisk together the flour, sugar, cocoa powder, egg replacer, baking soda, salt, and chopped nuts.
3. In a medium-sized bowl, mix together the cherries, soy milk, olive oil, and vanilla.
4. Using a spoon, combine the ingredients of the two bowls.
5. Pour batter into prepared pan(s).
6. Bake for 35 minutes or until toothpick inserted in the center of cake comes out clean.
7. Cool on counter for 10 minutes. Remove from pan(s) to wire cooling rack. Cool completely before frosting.
8. Frost if desired.

Dark sweet cherries make this moist cake a divine treat.

Carrot Cake

Yield: Two 8-inch rounds or one 9 x 13-inch cake

2 cups cake flour
1½ cups sugar
1 Tbs. egg replacer powder
2 tsp. baking powder
1½ tsp. cinnamon
¾ tsp. salt
½ tsp. nutmeg
1½ cups soy milk

¾ cup margarine
1 Tbs. vanilla
¾ cup shredded carrots
½ cup chopped walnuts
½ cup raisins
vanilla (p. 257) or maple (p. 256) frosting
    (optional)

* Preheat oven to 350°F.

1. Oil and flour pan(s).
2. In a large bowl, whisk together flour, sugar, egg replacer, baking powder, cinnamon, salt, and nutmeg.
3. Add soy milk, margarine, and vanilla. With an electric mixer, mix on low speed just until combined. Turn mixer to high and mix on high speed for 5 minutes.
4. Stir in the carrots, walnuts, and raisins.
5. Pour batter into prepared pan(s).
6. Bake for 35 minutes or until toothpick inserted in the center comes out clean.
7. Cool on counter for 10 minutes. Remove from pan(s) to wire cooling rack. Cool completely before frosting.
8. Frost if desired.

Chocolate Cake

Yield: Two 8-inch cake rounds or one 9 x 13-inch cake

1¾ cups + 2 Tbs. cake flour
¾ cup unsweetened baking cocoa powder
1½ tsp. baking soda
½ tsp. salt
2¼ tsp. egg replacer powder
3 Tbs. water

1⅗ cups unsweetened soy milk
¾ cup margarine
1½ cups sugar
¾ tsp. vanilla
½ tsp. almond extract
chocolate frosting (p. 253) (optional)

* Preheat oven to 350°F.

1. Oil and flour cake pan(s).
2. In a medium-sized bowl, mix flour, cocoa, baking soda, and salt.
3. In a separate bowl, whisk together egg replacer and water for 30 seconds, add soy milk, and whisk for 30 more seconds.
4. In a third bowl, beat margarine with electric mixer until softened.
5. Add sugar, vanilla, and almond extract to the margarine. Beat until well combined.
6. Add ½ of the liquid mixture to the margarine mixture and beat for 1 minute.
7. Add ½ of the flour mixture to the margarine mixture and beat for 1 minute.
8. Add remaining liquid mixture to the margarine mixture and beat for 1 minute.
9. Add remaining flour mixture to the margarine mixture and beat for 1½ minutes.
10. Pour cake batter into prepared pan(s).
11. Bake for 35 to 40 minutes or until toothpick inserted in center of cake comes out clean.
12. Cool on counter for 10 minutes. Remove from pan(s) to wire cooling rack. Cool completely before frosting.
13. Frost if desired.

Variation: CHOCOLATE CUPCAKES (Yield: 24 cupcakes)

Oil and flour muffin cups, or use paper baking cup liners. Fill cups ⅗ full with chocolate cake batter. Bake for 18–20 minutes at 350°F or until toothpick inserted in center comes out clean.

Variation: THREE 8-inch ROUNDS OF CHOCOLATE CAKE, OR 36 CUPCAKES

Increase ingredients to: 2½ cups cake flour, 1 cup unsweetened cocoa powder, 2 tsp. baking soda, ½ tsp. salt, 1 Tbs. egg replacer powder, ¼ cup water, 2¼ cups soy milk, 1 cup margarine, 2 cups sugar, 1 tsp. vanilla, and ¾ tsp. almond extract.

Coconut Cake

Two 8-inch white cake rounds, cooled (p. 252)
1 batch coconut frosting, cooled (p. 254)

1. Split each cake round in half, creating 4 layers of cake.
2. Stack each cake layer on top of each other with frosting separating each layer. Frost top of cake, but not the sides.
3. Keep refrigerated.

German Chocolate Cake

Yield: Two 8-inch round cakes

Two prepared 8-inch chocolate cakes (p. 248)
Prepared hazelnut coconut frosting (p. 255)

After chocolate cakes are baked and cooled, fill and frost with hazelnut coconut frosting.

Pineapple Upside Down Cake

Yield: 9 x 13-inch cake

One batch white cake batter (p. 252)
¾ cup brown sugar*
¼ cup extra light olive oil
1 16-oz. can pineapple rings, drained

*You can make your own brown sugar by combining ¾ cup sugar with 1 Tbs. molasses.

---

*   Preheat oven to 350°F.

1.   Pan spray a 9 x 13-inch baking dish.
2.   In a small bowl, combine brown sugar and oil.
3.   Evenly spread out sugar mixture on bottom of baking dish.
4.   Arrange pineapple evenly on top of sugar mixture.
5.   Gently pour cake batter over pineapple and sugar mixture.
6.   Bake 35 minutes or until toothpick inserted in center comes out clean.
7.   Cool on counter for 10 minutes.
8.   Loosen cake edges and invert cake onto cookie sheet while cake is still warm.
9.   Serve warm or cooled.

White Cake

Yield: Two 8-inch cake rounds or one 9 x 13-inch cake

3 cups cake flour
2 tsp. baking powder
½ tsp. salt
2 tsp. egg replacer powder
¼ cup water

1½ cups unsweetened soy milk
½ cup margarine
1⅓ cups sugar
1 Tbs. vanilla
vanilla frosting (p. 257) (optional)

*   Preheat oven to 350°F.

1. Oil and flour cake pan(s).
2. In a medium-sized bowl, mix flour, baking powder, and salt.
3. In a separate bowl, whisk together egg replacer and water for 30 seconds, add soy milk, and whisk for 30 more seconds.
4. In a third bowl, beat margarine with electric mixer until softened.
5. Add sugar and vanilla to the margarine. Beat until well combined.
6. Add ½ of the liquid mixture to the margarine mixture and beat for 1 minute.
7. Add ½ of the flour mixture to the margarine mixture and beat for 1 minute.
8. Add remaining liquid mixture to the margarine mixture and beat for 1 minute.
9. Add remaining flour mixture to the margarine mixture and beat for 1½ minutes.
10. Pour cake batter into prepared pan(s).
11. Bake for 28 to 32 minutes or until toothpick inserted in center of cake comes out clean.
12. Cool on counter for 10 minutes. Remove from pan(s) to wire cooling rack. Cool completely before frosting.
13. Frost if desired.

Variation: WHITE CUPCAKES (Yield: 24 cupcakes)
Oil and flour muffin cups, or use paper baking cup liners. Fill cups ⅔ full with cake batter. Bake for 18 to 20 minutes at 350°F or until toothpick inserted in center comes out clean.

Chocolate Frosting

Yield: Enough frosting for a double or triple layered 8-inch cake

3 Tbs. margarine
3 oz. unsweetened chocolate baking squares
3 cups powdered sugar
½ cup soy milk
1 tsp. vanilla

⅛ tsp. salt (optional)
ice water

1. In a double boiler, melt margarine and chocolate. Pour into a medium-sized bowl.
3. Add powdered sugar, soy milk, vanilla, and salt. Frosting will be thin.
4. Fill a large bowl ⅓ full of water and ice cubes.
5. Place the bowl of frosting into the ice water, making sure the ice water doesn't over-flow into the frosting bowl.
6. Beat frosting on medium speed with an electric mixer until frosting firms up and turns lighter in color.

Coconut Frosting

Yield: Enough frosting for a double layered 8-inch cake

½ cup sugar
2 Tbs. cornstarch
1 14-oz. can unsweetened coconut milk
1 cup soy milk
1 cup unsweetened coconut flakes

1. In a small bowl, thoroughly mix sugar and cornstarch.
2. Pour coconut milk and soy milk into a 3-quart saucepan and place over medium heat. Heat until almost boiling, stirring frequently.
3. Whisk the sugar mixture in the hot soy milk, stirring constantly. When mixture comes to a boil, continue cooking and stirring for 1 more minute.
4. Remove from heat and stir in coconut flakes.
5. Chill well before using.

Hazelnut Coconut Frosting

Yield: Enough frosting for a double layered 8-inch cake

1½ cups hazelnuts
1½ cups soy milk
¾ cup sugar
¾ cup unsweetened shredded coconut
1 Tbs. cornstarch
½ tsp. vanilla

* Preheat oven to 325°F.

1. Toast hazelnuts in oven for 8 minutes or until light brown.
2. Chop hazelnuts.
3. In a 3-quart saucepan, combine all ingredients.
4. Heat on medium heat until hot but not boiling, stirring constantly.
5. Chill.

Variation: WALNUT COCONUT FROSTING
Substitute walnuts for hazelnuts.

Great for German Chocolate Cake.

Maple Frosting

Yield: Enough frosting for a
double layered 8-inch cake

3 cups powdered sugar
⅓ cup margarine, softened
¼ cup pure maple syrup

In a medium-sized bowl, blend all ingredients with an electric mixer until smooth.

Great on carrot cake!

Vanilla Frosting

Yield: Enough frosting for a double layered 8-inch cake or 24 cupcakes

3 cups powdered sugar
⅓ cup margarine, softened
2 tsp. vanilla
2 Tbs. soy milk

1. In a medium-sized bowl, with an electric mixer, mix sugar, margarine, and vanilla.
2. Add soy milk and beat until smooth. Add additional soy milk if needed.

Banana Pudding

12⅓ oz. silken tofu (about 1½ cups)
3 ripe bananas, sliced
¼ cup sugar
1 tsp. vanilla

1. In a food processor, process tofu, sugar, and vanilla until smooth.
2. Transfer to a bowl and stir in bananas.
3. Chill.

Variation: NO SUGAR ADDED BANANA PUDDING
For sugar, substitute ¼ tsp. powdered stevia extract.

Chocolate Pudding

Yield: 6 servings

2 cups soy milk
1 cup silken tofu
1 cup sugar
2 oz. unsweetened baking chocolate squares
   (chopped)
¼ cup cornstarch

2 Tbs. unsweetened cocoa powder
1 Tbs. vanilla extract
¼ tsp. salt

1. In a blender, blend all ingredients.
2. Transfer to a 3-quart saucepan. Slowly bring to a boil, stirring constantly.
3. Remove from heat and chill in refrigerator, stirring occasionally.

Variation: REDUCED-SUGAR CHOCOLATE PUDDING
Reduce sugar to ½ cup and add ½ tsp. powdered stevia extract.

Instant Chocolate Pudding

Yield: 4 servings

16 oz. silken tofu
¾ cup sugar
½ cup unsweetened cocoa powder
2 Tbs. vanilla

1. In a food processor, process all ingredients until smooth.
2. Chill before serving.

Coconut Pudding

12⅓ oz. extra firm silken tofu (about 1½ cups)
1 14-oz. can unsweetened coconut milk
1 cup soy milk
¾ cup sugar

¼ cup cornstarch
⅗ cup unsweetened coconut flakes

1. In a blender, blend all ingredients, except coconut flakes, until smooth.
2. Transfer to a 3-quart saucepan. Slowly bring to a boil, stirring constantly.
3. Remove from heat and stir in coconut.
4. Chill pudding in refrigerator, stirring occasionally.

Variation: REDUCED-SUGAR COCONUT PUDDING
Reduce sugar to ¼ cup and add ½ tsp. powdered stevia extract.

Rice Pudding

Yield: 5 servings

2 cups 10-minute instant brown or white
    rice, uncooked
1¾ cups soy milk
1 cup water
⅓ cup sugar
⅓ Tbs. extra light olive oil

1 Tbs. vanilla
½ cup raisins
½ cup chopped walnuts

1. In a 3-quart saucepan, add rice, soy milk, water, sugar, oil, and vanilla. Bring to a boil, reduce heat to low, cover, and simmer for 15 minutes or until rice is tender.
2. Remove from heat. Stir in raisins and walnuts. Cover and let sit for 5 minutes.
3. Serve warm, or refrigerate and serve cold.

Variation: REDUCED-SUGAR RICE PUDDING
Reduce sugar to 3 Tbs. and add ⅛ tsp. powdered stevia extract.

Tapioca Pudding

Yield: 5 servings

½ cup quick-cooking tapioca
¾ cup sugar
4 cups soy milk
1 Tbs. cornstarch
1 Tbs. vanilla

1. In a 3-quart saucepan, combine all ingredients and let sit for 5 minutes.
2. On medium heat, slowly bring to a low boil, stirring constantly.
3. Remove from heat and chill in refrigerator, stirring occasionally.

Variation: MAPLE TAPIOCA PUDDING
For sugar, substitute ⅓ cup pure maple syrup.

Variation: REDUCED-SUGAR TAPIOCA PUDDING
Reduce sugar to ¼ cup and add ½ tsp. powdered stevia extract.

Vanilla Pudding

Yield: 4 servings

¼ cup sugar
3 Tbs. cornstarch
⅛ tsp. salt
2 cups unsweetened soy milk
2 Tbs. margarine
1 Tbs. vanilla

1. In a small bowl, thoroughly mix sugar, cornstarch, and salt.
2. Pour soy milk in a 3-quart saucepan and place over medium heat. Heat until almost boiling, stirring frequently.
3. Whisk the sugar mixture into the hot soy milk, stirring constantly. When mixture comes to a boil, continue cooking and stirring for 1 more minute.
4. Remove from heat and whisk in the margarine and vanilla.
5. Chill pudding in refrigerator, stirring occasionally.

Vanilla Tofu Pudding

Yield: 4 servings

3 cups soy milk
1½ cups silken tofu
¾ cup sugar
¼ cup cornstarch
2 Tbs. vanilla
⅛ tsp. salt

1. In a blender, blend all ingredients until smooth.
2. Transfer to a 3-quart saucepan. Slowly bring to a boil, stirring frequently.
3. Remove from heat and chill in refrigerator, stirring occasionally.

Variation: REDUCED-SUGAR VANILLA TOFU PUDDING
Reduce sugar by ¼ cup and add ½ tsp. powdered stevia extract.

Apple Crisp

5 cups peeled and cored apple slices
3 Tbs. sugar
¾ cup brown sugar
½ cup flour
⅗ cup quick-cooking oatmeal (uncooked)

½ tsp. cinnamon
⅓ cup margarine, softened

*   Preheat oven to 375°F.

1. In a medium-sized bowl, coat apple slices with 3 Tbs. sugar.
2. Pour apples into a lightly oiled 8 x 8-inch baking dish.
3. Mix remaining ingredients and sprinkle over apples.
4. Bake until topping is golden brown and apples start to bubble, about 30 minutes.

Serve warm with vegan vanilla ice cream if desired. You can use pears or peaches instead of apples if you'd like.

Baked Apples in Pastry

Yield: 4 servings

4 medium-sized baking apples
¼ cup sugar (brown or white)
¾ tsp. cinnamon
½ cup apple juice
4 tsp. margarine

1 single pie crust, divided into 4 pieces
 (p. 233)

* Preheat oven to 425°F.

1. Peel and core apples. A melon baller is excellent for removing the core of the apple. If you do not have a melon baller, use a small knife to remove the core, leaving the apple in one whole piece.
2. In a small bowl, mix sugar and cinnamon and set aside.
3. Roll one piece of pie crust into a ball and slightly flatten. Place dough between 2 pieces of waxed paper and roll out. Remove top layer of waxed paper. Place apple on center of dough. Bring dough up and around apple, leaving a hole at the top, trimming extra dough off if necessary. Pinch edges of pastry together so the filling will not leak out. Repeat with remaining apples.
4. Place apples (without waxed paper) in a baking dish.
5. Fill each apple with 1 Tbs. sugar mixture, 2 Tbs. apple juice, and 1 tsp. margarine.
6. Bake 45 minutes or until pastry is lightly browned, juice is bubbling, and apple is tender.

Serve warm with vegan vanilla ice cream.

Baklava

2¼ cups finely chopped walnuts
3 Tbs. brown sugar
1 cup sugar
¾ cup water
¼ cup pure maple syrup
3 Tbs. lemon juice

¼ tsp. cinnamon
16 oz. phyllo dough (20 whole sheets or 40 half sheets*), thawed in refrigerator overnight
¾ cup margarine, melted

* A half sheet of phyllo dough is usually the same size as a 9 x 13-inch baking dish.

1. Combine walnuts and brown sugar. Set walnut mixture aside.
2. In a medium-sized saucepan, bring sugar, water, maple syrup, lemon juice, and cinnamon to a boil. Reduce heat to low and simmer for 10 minutes. Cool to room temperature.
3. Lightly oil a 9 x 13-inch baking dish.
4. If using 20 full sheets, cut them in half so you now have 40 half sheets, the size of your 9 x 13-inch baking dish. Divide into 4 even stacks of 10 sheets each (if your package of phyllo dough has extra sheets, go ahead and use them by dividing them among your 4 stacks.) Cover each stack with clear wrap.
5. Place one sheet of phyllo dough in baking dish and very lightly brush with some of the melted margarine. Repeat until first stack of dough is used, brushing each sheet with margarine.
6. Top with a third of the walnut mixture.
7. Repeat steps 4 and 5, ending with a layer of phyllo dough that is generously brushed with melted margarine.
8. Cover and refrigerate for 15 minutes.
9. Preheat oven to 325°F.
10. Remove baklava from refrigerator. Precut baklava (still in baking dish) into 36 pieces, being sure to cut all the way through to the bottom.
11. Bake for 45 minutes.
12. Remove from oven and immediately pour the cool syrup evenly over the top.
13. Let cool completely. Cut again, if needed.

Variation: ALMOND BAKLAVA
Substitute almonds for the walnuts.

Berry Crisp

Yield: 6 servings

4 cups fresh blackberries or other berries*   ½ tsp. cinnamon
¾ cup brown sugar   ⅓ cup margarine, softened
½ cup flour
⅗ cup quick cooking oats (uncooked)

*If berries are a bit sour, you can gently toss them with sugar to taste.

*   Preheat oven to 375°F.

1.   Place berries in a lightly oiled 8 x 8-inch baking dish.
2.   Mix remaining ingredients and sprinkle over berries.
3.   Bake until topping is golden brown and berries are bubbling, about 25 minutes.

**Serve warm with vegan vanilla
ice cream if desired.**

Brownies

1 cup flour*
¾ cup cocoa powder
1¼ cups sugar
⅛ tsp. baking powder
½ tsp. salt
¾ cup chocolate chips

¼ cup chopped walnuts (optional)
⅓ cup soy milk
⅓ cup extra light olive oil
¼ cup silken tofu
1 Tbs. vanilla

*You can use half white flour and half whole wheat flour if you prefer.

* Preheat oven to 350°F.

1. In large bowl, whisk together flour, cocoa powder, sugar, baking powder, salt, walnuts, and chocolate chips.
2. In a blender, blend the soy milk, oil, tofu, and vanilla.
3. Add blended mixture to the flour mixture in the large bowl and stir until just combined. Batter will be thick.
4. Spread batter out evenly into an 8 x 8-inch oiled baking dish.
5. Bake for 35 minutes or until toothpick inserted in the middle comes out clean.

Rich chocolate brownies.

Chocolate-Dipped Strawberries

Yield: 24 large dipped strawberries

24 strawberries with stems (rinsed and patted dry)
1 cup chocolate chips
1 oz. unsweetened chocolate baking squares
¼ cup soy milk

1. Place chocolate chips, chocolate squares, and soy milk in a double boiler.
2. Slowly heat until just melted, stirring occasionally.
3. Remove from heat but leave in double boiler to keep chocolate sauce soft for dipping.
4. Dip strawberries into melted chocolate and place on waxed paper to cool.
5. Refrigerate, uncovered, for 30 minutes, to allow chocolate to set.
6. Keep in refrigerator until ready to serve.

Variation: CHOCOLATE-DIPPED MARZIPAN
For the strawberries, substitute pieces of marzipan.

Fruit Cobbler

Filling:
4 cups fresh, canned, or frozen (thawed)
    fruit (peaches, plums, assorted berries,
    cherries, etc.)
½ cup water
½ cup sugar
1 Tbs. lemon juice
3 Tbs. cornstarch
½ tsp. cinnamon (optional)

Dumplings:
1 cup flour
1 Tbs. sugar
1½ tsp. baking powder
½ tsp. salt
3 Tbs. extra light olive oil
½ cup soy milk

* Preheat oven to 400°F.

1. In a 3-quart saucepan, combine fruit, water, sugar, lemon juice, cornstarch, and cinnamon.
2. Cook over medium heat, stirring constantly, until mixture comes to a boil and thickens.
3. Transfer fruit to an 8 x 8-inch baking dish.
4. In a medium-sized bowl, whisk together the flour, 1 Tbs. sugar, baking powder, and salt.
5. With a spoon, stir in the oil and milk. Stir just until combined.
6. Drop 6 dumplings on top of the fruit mixture.
7. Bake, uncovered, for 25 minutes or until toothpick inserted in the center of a dumpling comes out clean.

Fruit Danish

Yield: 25 pastries

1 Tbs. dry yeast (¼-oz. package)
¼ cup + 1 Tbs. sugar
1 cup warm water (110°F)
2½ cups flour
⅓ cup light olive oil

1 tsp. salt
¼ tsp. vanilla
1 12-oz. canned fruit pie filling (cherry, blueberry, etc.)
2 Tbs. extra light olive oil

1. In a large bowl, whisk together the yeast, 1 Tbs. sugar, and warm water. Let stand for 5 minutes.
2. Add the flour, ⅓ cup oil, ¼ cup sugar, salt, and vanilla.
3. On a floured surface, knead dough for 3 minutes.
4. Place dough in a large oiled bowl, cover with a slightly damp towel, and let stand in a warm place until doubled in size, about 1½ hours.
5. Punch down dough and knead for 1 minute.
6. On a floured surface, roll out dough to 15 x 20 inches.
7. Cut into 3 x 4-inch pieces. Place 2 Tbs. fruit filling in center of each square.
8. Fold two opposite corners together so they overlap. Place on a lightly oiled baking sheet. Let stand for 20 minutes.
9. Preheat oven to 350°F.
10. Bake pastries for 12 minutes. Lightly brush pastries with 2 Tbs. oil and continue to cook for 5 more minutes or until pastry is no longer doughy in center.

A sweet fruit-filled pastry.

Fruit Tart

Yield: 8 servings

Single citrus pie crust (p. 235)
⅓ batch vanilla pudding, chilled (p. 264)
⅓ cup apple jelly
3 cups cut-up assorted fresh fruit (strawberries, peaches, mango, kiwi, or blueberries)

1. Place citrus crust in a 9-inch tart or pie dish. Bake for 10 minutes in a preheated 375°F oven. Cool.
2. Pour pudding in cooled pie crust.
3. Neatly arrange fruit on top of pudding.
4. In a 2-quart saucepan, slowly heat jelly until it turns to a liquid.
5. Evenly pour melted jelly on top of fruit.
6. Chill tart, uncovered, in refrigerator for 30 minutes.

Grandma's Caramel Corn

Yield: 3 quarts

½ cup margarine
½ cup brown sugar
2 Tbs. light corn syrup
½ tsp. salt
¼ baking soda

½ tsp. vanilla
12 cups popped corn

*   Preheat oven to 250°F.

1.   Oil a 9 x 13-inch baking dish.
2.   Place popped corn in the dish.
3.   In a 2-quart saucepan, add the margarine, brown sugar, corn syrup, and salt. Bring to a boil, stirring constantly. Reduce heat to low and let simmer for 5 minutes without stirring.
4.   Remove from heat and stir in baking soda and vanilla. Immediately pour over popped corn and stir well to coat all pieces.
5.   Spread out evenly in baking dish.
6.   Bake, uncovered, for 1 hour, gently stirring every 15 minutes.
7.   Cool and break apart.

Variation: CARAMEL CORN WITH PEANUTS
Add 1 cup Spanish, Virginia, or dry roasted peanuts to popcorn before adding syrup.

Pecan Pie Squares

Yield: 32 small squares

Filling:
3½ cups finely chopped toasted pecans
1¼ cups sugar
¾ tsp. cornstarch or arrowroot
1½ tsp. vanilla
⅗ cup water

⅛ tsp. salt
Single pie crust, uncooked (p. 233)

*   **Preheat oven to 425°F.**

1. Thoroughly combine all filling ingredients.
2. Prepare pie crust. Roll out dough between sheets of waxed paper or on a lightly floured surface to fit a 9 x 13-inch baking dish. Place pastry in baking dish.
3. Spread filling evenly over the pastry.
4. Bake for 20 minutes or until pie crust is very lightly browned.
5. Cool before serving. Do a 4 x 8 cut to get 32 small squares.

> **This dessert makes a great appetizer; the small squares are just right for nibbling on while your party gets underway.**

Strawberry Short Cakes

Yield: 8 servings

2 cups flour*
2 Tbs. sugar
1 Tbs. baking powder
1 tsp. salt
¾ cup soy milk

⅓ cup extra light olive oil
2 pints strawberries, sliced (sweetened with
    sugar, if desired)
1 quart vegan vanilla ice cream

*You can use half white flour and half whole wheat flour if you prefer.

1. In a medium-sized bowl, whisk together flour, sugar, baking powder and salt.
2. Stir in the milk and oil just until combined.
3. Turn dough out onto a lightly floured surface and knead 10 times.
4. Roll out to ½-inch thickness.
5. Cut into 8 pieces.
6. Place 1 inch apart on ungreased cookie sheet.
7. Bake 10 to 12 minutes or until lightly browned.
8. While still warm, split cakes in half crosswise and serve with berries and vanilla soy ice cream.

Variation: FRUIT SHORT CAKES

For the strawberries, substitute other fresh fruits, such as blueberries, bananas, or peaches.

Whipped "Cream"

12⅓ oz. extra firm silken tofu (about 1½ cups)
1 cup sugar
¼ cup water
2 tsp. vanilla

In a blender or food processor, combine all ingredients until smooth.

Miscellaneous

(Gravies, Sauces, Spreads, Tofu, Other)

Country Gravy

Yield: 3 cups

¼ cup light olive oil
⅓ cup flour
2½ cups soy milk
2 tsp. onion powder
salt to taste (about 1 tsp.)
pepper to taste (about ½ tsp.)

1. In a 2-quart saucepan, combine oil and flour. Cook on medium/low heat for 2 minutes, stirring constantly.
2. Add soy milk and onion powder. Increase heat to medium.
3. Heat until hot and thickened, stirring frequently.
4. Add salt and pepper to taste.

Serve over potatoes or biscuits.

Mushroom Gravy

Yield: 1½ cups

6 mushrooms, sliced
1½ Tbs. light olive oil
1½ Tbs. flour
¼ tsp. thyme
¾ cup soy milk

¼ cup vegetable broth
salt to taste (about ½ tsp.)

1. In a 2-quart saucepan, sauté mushrooms in oil until tender. Reduce heat to low.
2. On reduced heat, add flour and thyme. Sauté 3 minutes.
3. Add soy milk and vegetable broth. Increase heat to medium.
4. Bring to a low boil, stirring frequently.
5. Add salt to taste.

Sage Gravy

¼ cup light olive oil
⅓ cup flour
1 tsp. sage
½ tsp. thyme
¼ cup nutritional yeast flakes (optional)

3 cups vegetable broth
salt to taste (about ½ tsp.)

1. In a 3-quart saucepan, combine the oil, flour, sage, and thyme. Cook on stove top at medium/low heat for 2 minutes, stirring constantly.
2. Add vegetable broth and nutritional yeast flakes. Increase heat to medium.
3. Cook until thickened, stirring frequently.
4. Add salt to taste.

Excellent with mashed potatoes and vegan turkey!

Blueberry Sauce

Yield: 2½ cups

3 Tbs. cornstarch
¼ cup sugar
½ cup water
1 16 oz. bag frozen blueberries

1. In a small bowl, thoroughly mix cornstarch and sugar.
2. In a 3-quart saucepan, combine water and blueberries. Over medium heat, cook until blueberries are thawed and can be easily stirred.
3. While stirring, add the cornstarch and sugar mixture to the blueberries and water.
4. Continue to cook until hot and thickened, stirring constantly.

Variation: REDUCED-SUGAR BLUEBERRY SAUCE

Reduce sugar to 2 Tbs. and add ⅛ tsp. powdered stevia extract.

Variation: NO SUGAR ADDED BLUEBERRY SAUCE

For sugar, substitute ¼ tsp. powdered stevia extract.

Use this sauce on top of pancakes, waffles, crepes, and ice cream.

"Cheese" Sauce

Yield: 2½ cups

2 cups soy milk
2 Tbs. light olive oil
¼ cup flour
1 2-oz. jar pimientos
½ cup yeast flakes
2 Tbs. peanut, almond, or soy butter

½ tsp. garlic (optional)
½ tsp. paprika
1½ tsp. salt

1. In a blender, blend all ingredients, except salt, until smooth.
2. Pour sauce into a 3-quart saucepan.
3. On medium heat, heat sauce until hot and thickened, stirring frequently.
4. Add salt to taste.

Variation: NACHO "CHEESE" SAUCE
Increase garlic to 1 teaspoon, substitute chili powder for paprika, and add one 4-oz. can of diced green chilies.

Great with baked potatoes or vegetables.

Peanut Sauce

½ cup peanut butter
¼ cup sesame oil
2 Tbs. soy sauce*

2 Tbs. water
⅛ tsp. cayenne pepper (optional)

*Substitute Bragg liquid aminos if you prefer.

In a small bowl, combine all ingredients.

Peanut sauce can be used as sauce for stir-fries, a spread for wraps, or a dip for spring rolls.

Pesto

Yield: 1 cup

2 bunches fresh basil, stemmed and
    chopped
⅓ cup light olive oil
1 head of fresh garlic, peeled (about 16
    cloves)
½ cup pine nuts

salt to taste (about 1½ tsp.)

Place basil, olive oil, garlic, and pine nuts in a food processor and process until smooth.
Add salt to taste.

You can use roasted
garlic in this recipe for
a smoother flavor.

Pizza Sauce

Yield: Enough sauce for 1 large or 2 medium pizzas

6 oz. tomato paste
1 tsp. basil
1 tsp. oregano
½ tsp. garlic* (optional)

¾ tsp. salt
2 Tbs. water
1 Tbs. light olive oil

*Substitute onion powder if you prefer.

In a small bowl, whisk together all ingredients.

A rich flavored pizza sauce.

Sun-dried Tomato Pizza Sauce

Yield: Enough sauce for one medium pizza

10 sun-dried tomatoes
½ onion, diced
½ cup water
2 Tbs. light olive oil
2 tsp. sugar
1 tsp. salt

½ tsp. garlic (optional)
½ tsp. basil

1. In a 2-quart saucepan, add all ingredients.
2. Over medium heat, bring to a boil, reduce heat to low, cover, and simmer for 10 minutes.
3. Pour into a blender and blend until smooth.

Stir-fry Sauce

Yield: 2 cups

¾ cup sugar
2 Tbs. cornstarch
1 cup cold water
¼ cup soy sauce*
¼ cup seasoned rice vinegar

1 Tbs. sesame oil
½ tsp. garlic
¼ tsp. ginger
pinch of red pepper flakes (optional)

*Substitute Bragg liquid aminos if desired.

1. In a 3-quart saucepan, combine all ingredients.
2. Over medium heat, cook until thickened, stirring frequently.

Use this sauce for stir-fries or as a dipping sauce.

Caramelized Onion & Garlic Spread

Yield: 1 cup

1 small sweet onion, diced
8 cloves fresh garlic, peeled
3 Tbs. light olive oil
salt to taste (about ½ tsp.)

1. In a 2-quart saucepan, on medium/low heat, sauté the onion and garlic in the oil until onions are a nice deep brown color.
2. Place sautéed onions and garlic in a food processor and process until smooth.
3. Add salt to taste.

A flavorful spread you can use as a pizza sauce or on a sandwich.

Pesto Mayonnaise

Yield: 1 cup

¼ cup pesto (p. 286)
¾ cup vegan mayonnaise

In a small bowl, combine pesto and mayonnaise. Keep refrigerated.

Roasted Vegetable "Cream Cheese" Spread

Yield: 1½ cups

1 small sweet onion, diced
1 red bell pepper, diced
2 cloves garlic, peeled and diced
3 Tbs. light olive oil
½ tsp. basil

1 8-oz. tub vegan cream cheese
salt to taste (about ¼ tsp.)

*   **Preheat oven to 475°F.**

1.   In a small bowl, toss the onion, pepper, garlic, oil, and basil together.
2.   Transfer to an 8 x 8-inch baking dish.
3.   Bake, uncovered, for 20 minutes or until vegetables are browned.
4.   Chill roasted vegetables in refrigerator.
5.   Place roasted vegetables and cream cheese in a food processor and process until smooth.
6.   Add salt to taste.

This spread can be used as a dip or as a sandwich spread.

Marinated Grilled Tofu

Yield: 3 servings

---

1 pound pressed tofu (p. 294)

Marinade:
¼ cup soy sauce*
2 Tbs. light olive oil

*Substitute Bragg liquid aminos if desired.

½ tsp. garlic
½ tsp. onion powder
½ tsp. thyme
½ tsp. basil

---

1. In a small bowl, combine soy sauce, oil, garlic, onion powder, thyme, and basil.
2. Marinate pressed tofu for 1–2 hours in the refrigerator.
3. Heat grill or skillet to 375°F.
4. Drain off marinade and grill each side of tofu until lightly browned.

Variation: LEMON THYME MARINATED GRILLED TOFU

Marinade: In a blender, blend ¼ cup chopped onion, 1 tsp. garlic, 1 tsp. salt, 1 tsp. thyme, ½ tsp. basil, ¼ tsp. chili pepper flakes, ¼ cup lemon juice, ¼ cup light olive oil, and ¼ cup water.

> **Marinated tofu can be cooled and used in salads, or kept hot and served with rice and a sauce.**

Pressed Tofu

Yield: 3 servings

16 oz. firm or extra firm tofu

1. Drain and rinse tofu.
2. Slice tofu into 3 thinner slabs.
3. On a cookie sheet, spread out tofu pieces between two dry towels.
4. Place a second cookie sheet on top of the top towel.
5. Place a heavy object on top of the second cookie sheet. A large pot filled with water works well.
6. Press for 30 minutes.

Press tofu when you want a firmer, drier tofu, well suited for marinating and grilling.

Teriyaki Tofu

Yield: 3 servings

16 oz. pressed tofu, large dice (p. 294)
2 Tbs. soy sauce*
1 Tbs. sesame oil

*Substitute Bragg liquid aminos if desired.

---

*   **Preheat oven to 375°F.**

1. In a small bowl, toss pressed tofu with soy sauce and oil.
2. Place tofu evenly on a cookie sheet.
3. Bake uncovered for 30 minutes.

Variation: SESAME SEED–ENCRUSTED TOFU
Add 2 Tbs. sesame seeds while tossing tofu.

Teriyaki tofu can be served hot with a stir-fry or cold with a salad.

Crepes

2 cups flour
3 Tbs. sugar
2 Tbs. baking powder
1 tsp. salt
12⅓ oz. silken tofu (about 1½ cups)
3 cups soy milk

½ cup extra light olive oil
1 Tbs. vanilla
pan spray

* **Preheat griddle to 400°F, or choose the medium heat setting on your stove.**

1. In a large bowl, whisk together flour, sugar, baking powder, and salt.
2. In a blender, blend tofu, soy milk, oil, and vanilla.
3. Whisk together the blended ingredients with the flour mixture.
4. Pan spray the griddle. Pour one quarter of the batter down the center of the griddle. Spread batter out evenly over the entire griddle.
5. When crepes are browned on the underside, make three cuts to divide crepes into 4 pieces. Flip crepes and cook for 2 more minutes. Roll up crepes, and place cooked crepes on a cookie sheet, in a 170° oven, to keep warm while you finish cooking the remaining crepes.

Croutons

1 pound fresh sourdough bread, cubed
3 Tbs. parsley flakes
2 Tbs. basil
1 Tbs. garlic
1 Tbs. onion powder
1 Tbs. thyme

1 tsp. oregano
1 tsp. salt
½ tsp. paprika
¼ tsp. black pepper
⅓ cup light olive oil

* **Preheat oven to 375°F.**

1. In a large bowl, stir together the parsley, basil, garlic, onion powder, thyme, oregano, salt, paprika, and pepper.
2. Add the bread cubes and toss until coated with spices.
3. Stir in the olive oil (your hands work well on this step).
4. Divide croutons between 2 cookie sheets.
5. Bake for 20 minutes, stirring once after 10 minutes. Rotate pans from top to bottom and bottom to top after 10 minutes for even cooking, if needed.
6. Cool, uncovered.
7. Store in an airtight container.

Homemade croutons have a nice fresh taste.

Parmesan "Cheese"

Yield: 2 cups

8 oz. sliced almonds
¼ cup nutritional yeast flakes
¼ cup basil
2 Tbs. onion powder
1 Tbs. garlic
1 Tbs. oregano

1 Tbs. dried lemon peel
1 tsp. salt
½ tsp. paprika
¼ tsp. nutmeg

1. Place all ingredients in a food processor and process well.
2. Store in a sealed container in the refrigerator.

Sprinkle on top of pasta, salads, or soups.

Toasted Coconut

Yield: ¼ cup

¼ cup coconut flakes

*   Preheat oven to 350°F.

1.   Spread out coconut on a cookie sheet.
2.   Bake for 5 minutes or until lightly browned. (Freshly shredded coconut will take longer to brown than packaged coconut flakes.)

Variation: TOASTED SLIVERED OR SLICED ALMONDS
For coconut, substitute slivered almonds and bake for 7 minutes.

Variation: TOASTED SESAME SEEDS
For coconut, substitute sesame seeds and bake for 7 minutes.

Vegetable Broth

Yield: 4 cups

3 cups chopped carrots
3 cups chopped celery
3 cups chopped onions
2 tomatoes, diced
1 bunch parsley, chopped

2 bay leaves
1 tsp. thyme

1. Place all ingredients in a large pot.
2. Add water so it just covers the vegetables.
3. Bring to a boil, reduce heat to low, cover, and simmer for 2 hours.
4. Strain out vegetables, keeping the liquid and discarding the vegetables.
5. Place vegetable broth back in the pot, bring to a low boil, and cook, uncovered, until liquid is reduced to 4 cups.

You can save your vegetable trimmings in the freezer until you have enough for a batch of broth. You can also use other vegetables than the ones mentioned here.

Cook's Notes

- Be sure to wash all produce before using.
- Light olive oil is light in color and flavor. It works well for baking and sautéing. Extra light olive oil or canola oil can be substituted for light olive oil.
- When a recipe calls for flour, use all-purpose white flour unless otherwise noted. You can use whole wheat flour (or half whole wheat flour) on any recipe, but it will have a heavier flavor and texture.
- Cookbook recipes were made with table salt. If using kosher salt, you may need to increase the amount.
- All herbs and spices are dry, unless otherwise noted.
- The sugar I use is evaporated cane juice. I have created reduced-sugar versions of several recipes using the natural sweetener stevia.

Glossary

Active dry yeast: A leavening agent used in baking.

Blend: To thoroughly mix.

Bulgur: Toasted cracked wheat.

Chill: To cool in a refrigerator until cold.

Chop: To cut into pieces with no consistent size or shape needed.

Couscous: A pasta, smaller than rice, made of semolina from durum wheat flour.

Cream: To thoroughly mix ingredients with a mixer, food processor, or several strokes with a wooden spoon.

Dice: To cut into ¼-inch x ¼-inch pieces. "Large dice" refers to foods cut into ½-inch x ½-inch pieces. "Small dice" refers to foods cut into ⅛-inch x ⅛-inch pieces.

Double boiler: A cooking utensil consisting of two pots that fit one on top of the other. Food is placed in the upper pot and water is boiled in the lower pot. Double boilers are used when food items should not be placed directly on heat.

Egg replacer: Made by Ener-G Foods. This is a powder that is used to help foods rise. Not to be confused with liquid egg substitute.

Garbanzo beans: Also known as chick peas.

Habanero: The hottest known chili, which is about the size of a walnut. The orange variety has a Scovilla unit rating of 210,000, while the red ones top out at 150,000.

Jalapeño: A finger-sized green or red chili that is popular in salsas. It can be found canned or fresh. It has a Scovilla unit rating of 25,000.

Julienne: To cut into ¼-inch strips.

Julienne, thin cut: To cut into ⅛-inch strips.

Knead: The process of pressing and folding dough until smooth and elastic. Kneading strengthens gluten strands so they can hold in the gas bubbles better.

Liquid aminos: A liquid protein concentrate made from soybeans, tasting similar to soy sauce. Made by Bragg.

Marinate: To soak an item in a savory sauce, called a marinade, to add flavor.

Mince: To cut into very small pieces.

Miso: Fermented soybean paste. Sold in the refrigerated section.

Nutritional yeast flakes: An inactive yeast that has no leavening agent and has a cheesy flavor. High in B vitamins and protein.

Pinch: ¹⁄₁₆ of a teaspoon.

Polenta: Course ground cornmeal. Also know as grits.

Puree: To process a food with a blender or food processor until smooth.

Roast: To cook in an oven, usually at a high temperature of 375°F or hotter.

Sauté: Rapid cooking done in an open pan on medium/high to high heat using minimal oil.

Semolina flour: A yellow flour made from durum wheat. It is high in gluten and protein.

Serrano: A thin 2-inch chili that is often used in Mexican cooking. It has a Scovilla unit rating of 4,000.

Sesame butter: Another name for tahini. Made from ground sesame seeds.

Shred: To cut into thin short strips. Usually done with a box grater or food processor with a grater attachment.

Simmer: To cook at a low temperature in order to allow flavors to blend.

Stevia: A calorie-free natural sweetener, made from the plant *Stevia rebaudiana*. It has been used for centuries and is up to 300 times sweeter than sugar.

Tahini: Also called sesame butter. Made from ground sesame seeds.

Toast: To brown in an oven or in a dry skillet.

Tofu, firm: A firm-textured tofu used for dicing, pressing, marinating, grilling, and roasting. Sold packed in water.

Tofu, pressed: Tofu that has been pressed in order to make it firmer and less moist.

Tofu, silken: A very smooth tofu used in baking and beverages. Available in water packs and aseptic packaging.

Vital wheat gluten: The naturally occurring protein in wheat. Can be found in packages or sold in bulk.

Whisk: To mix ingredients using a wire whip called a whisk.

White flour: Flour that has had the bran and germ removed.

Whole wheat flour: Flour ground using the whole grain, including the bran and germ.

Zest: The very outer rind of any citrus fruit, not including the inner white of the rind. Zest can be removed with a sharp knife, grater, or zester.

Conversion Chart

Measurement Conversions:

3 teaspoons = 1 tablespoon

6 teaspoons = 2 tablespoons = ⅛ cup

12 teaspoons = 4 tablespoons = ¼ cup

8 tablespoons = ½ cup

16 tablespoons = 1 cup

1 cup = ½ pint

2 cups = 1 pint

4 cups = 2 pints = 1 quart

8 cups = 4 pints = 2 quarts = ½ gallon

16 cups = 8 pints = 4 quarts = 1 gallon

Liquid volume conversions:

½ ounce = 1 tablespoon

1 ounce = ⅛ cup

2 ounces = ¼ cup

4 ounces = ½ cup

6 ounces = ¾ cup

8 ounces = 1 cup

16 ounces = 1 pint

32 ounces = 1 quart

64 ounces = ½ gallon

128 ounces = 1 gallon

Abbreviations:

Teaspoon: tsp.

Tablespoon: Tbs.

Ounce: oz.

Fluid ounce: fl. oz.

Pint: pt.

Quart: qt.

Gallon: gal.

A Well-Stocked Vegan Pantry

Baking:

Baking powder
Baking soda
Chocolate baking squares, unsweetened
Chocolate chips
Cocoa powder, unsweetened
Coconut flakes, unsweetened
Cornstarch
Egg replacer
Extracts:
  almond
  coconut
  maple
  rum
  vanilla
Flour:
  semolina
  white
  whole wheat
  vital wheat gluten
Olive oil:
  extra light
  light
Margarine

Molasses
Poppy seeds
Raisins
Salt
Stevia extract powder
Sugar:
  brown
  granulated
  powdered
Tapioca
Yeast, dry active

Dry goods:

Beans, assorted dried
Bran:
  oat
  wheat
Bulgur
Coconut milk, unsweetened
Cornmeal
Couscous
Farina
Flax seed

Kamut

Lentils:

  green

  red

Nutritional yeast flakes

Nuts:

  almonds

  filberts

  pecans

  walnuts

Oatmeal

Pan spray

Pasta:

  macaroni

  penne

  rotini

  spaghetti

Polenta, uncooked

Popcorn kernels

Rice:

  basmati

  brown

  calrose

  jasmine

  wild

Sesame oil

Soy sauce

Sun-dried tomatoes

Vegetable broth

Vinegar:

  apple cider

  balsamic

  red wine

  rice

Spices:

Allspice

Aniseed

Basil

Black pepper

Cardamom pods

Cayenne pepper

Chili powder

Cinnamon

Cloves, ground

Cloves, whole

Cream of tartar

Cumin

Curry

Curry paste:

  green

  red

Garam masala

Garlic

Ginger

Nutmeg

Onion powder

Oregano

Paprika

Parsley flakes

Red pepper flakes

Rosemary, ground

Sage
Sesame seeds
Thyme
Turmeric

Artichoke hearts
Baked beans
Beans:
    black
    garbanzo
    kidney
    pinto
Green chilies, diced
Olives
Pimientos, diced
Pineapple
Pumpkin
Refried beans
Split peas
Tomato:
    crushed
    diced
    paste
    sauce
Water chestnuts

Freezer items:
Blueberries
Corn

Green beans
Mangoes
Peas
Phyllo dough
Soybeans, shelled
Spinach

Refrigerator items:
Almond butter
Cheese (vegan), cheddar
Cheese (vegan), parmesan
Italian dressing
Lemon juice
Lime juice
Liquid aminos
Mayonnaise (vegan)
Miso
Mustard:
    Dijon
    yellow
Nondairy beverage:
    rice
    soy
Peanut butter
Relish:
    dill
    sweet
Salsa
Sesame butter (tahini)

Sweet chili sauce
Sweet relish
Tofu:
    firm
    ready-to-serve
    silken
Tortillas:
    corn
    flour
Worcestershire sauce (vegan)

Fresh produce:
Bell peppers
Carrots
Celery
Cilantro
Fruit
Garlic
Ginger
Lettuce
Mushrooms
Onions
Potatoes
Tomatoes

Miscellaneous items:
Cheesecloth
Clear wrap
Waxed paper

Protein List

Raw nuts & seeds: (1/4 cup, shelled)
Almonds...7g
Brazil nuts 5g
Cashews..4g
Coconut (shredded)........................2g
Filberts/hazelnuts 5g
Flax seeds 5g
Macadamia nuts 2g
Peanuts 8g
Pecans...2g
Pine nuts...4g
Pistachio nuts 6g
Pumpkin seeds................................7g
Sesame seeds 7g
Soy nuts...10g
Sunflower seeds 8g
Walnuts 5g

Beans: (1 cup cooked)
Adzuki beans 17g
Black beans.....................................15g
Black-eyed peas 14g
Cannellini 17g
Cranberry beans 17g

Fava beans 13g
Garbanzos (chick peas)...................15g
Great northern beans......................15g
Green peas (whole).........................9g
Kidney beans 15g
Lentils 18g
Lima beans 15g
Mung beans.....................................14g
Navy beans 16g
Pinto beans.....................................12g
Soybeans 29g
Split peas 16g

Soy products
Tempeh (4 oz)..................................12–20g
Textured vegetable protein (¼ cup)...10–12g
Tofu, extra firm (3 oz).....................7–12g
Tofu, firm (3 oz) 7–12g
Tofu, silken (3 oz)...........................4–6g

Grains (1/4 cup cooked)
Amaranth 7g
Barley, pearled 4–5g

Buckwheat groats 5–6g
Cornmeal (fine ground) 3g
Cornmeal (polenta, coarse) 3g
Millet, hulled 8.4g
Oat, bran 7g
Quinoa 5g
Rice, brown...................................3–5g
Rice, white 4g
Rice, wild......................................7g
Spelt, berries 6g
Wheat, bulgur................................5–6g
Wheat, whole berries......................6–9g

Nut butters (2 Tbs.)

Almond 5–8g
Cashew..4–5g
Peanut...5–6g
Sesame (tahini)..............................6g
Soy nut 6–7g

Milk substitutes (1 cup)

Almond 1–2g
Soy, lowfat/nonfat..........................4g
Soy, regular 6–9g
Multigrain 5g
Oat 4g
Rice 1g

Miscellaneous foods

Farina (¼ cup dry)..........................5g

Flour, rye (¼ cup) 4g
Flour, white unbleached (¼ cup) 4g
Flour, whole wheat (¼ cup) 5g
Kamut (¼ cup, cooked)...................5g
Kashi (½ cup, cooked) 6g
Oatmeal, quick (½ cup dry)............6g
Popcorn, yellow (¼ cup, kernels)......4g
Vital wheat gluten (¼ cup) 21g
Yeast flakes, nutritional (3 Tbs.) 8g
Yeast powder, nutritional (3 tsp.) 8g

Fresh vegetables*

Artichoke (medium).......................4g
Asparagus (5 spears).......................2g
Beans, string (1 cup) 2g
Beets (½ cup).................................1g
Broccoli (½ cup) 2g
Brussels sprouts (½ cup) 2g
Cabbage (½ cup)............................1g
Carrots (½ cup) 1g
Cauliflower (½ cup)........................1g
Celery (1 cup)................................1g
Chard, Swiss (1 cup).......................3g
Collards (1 cup) 4g
Corn, sweet (1 large cob) 5g
Cucumber* (1 cup) 1g
Eggplant (1 cup)............................1g
Fennel (1 medium bulb) 3g
Kale (1 cup) 2½g
Kohlrabi (1 cup) 3g

Leeks (1 cup) 1g
Lettuce* (1 cup) 1g
Okra (1 cup) 1g
Onion (½ cup) 1g
Parsnip (½ cup) 1g
Peas (½ cup) 4g
Peppers, bell (½ cup).......................1g
Potato, baked (2⅓ x 4¾") 5g
Radish (1 cup) 1g
Rhubarb (1 cup) 1g
Rutabaga (1 cup) 2g
Spinach* (1 cup) 1g
Squash, summer (1 cup) 2g
Squash, winter (1 cup) 2g
Sweet potato (1 cup).......................3g
Tomato* (1 medium) 1g
Turnip (1 cup) 1g

*All amounts refer to cooked vegetables except starred items, which are raw.

Index